SOUND BODY/
SOUND MIND

POTENTIALS
GUIDES FOR PRODUCTIVE LIVING

Wayne E. Oates, General Editor

SOUND BODY/ SOUND MIND

by
ALBERT L. MEIBURG

THE WESTMINSTER PRESS
Philadelphia

Copyright © 1984 Albert L. Meiburg

Book design by Alice Derr

First edition

Published by The Westminster Press®
Philadelphia, Pennsylvania

PRINTED IN THE UNITED STATES OF AMERICA
2   4   6   8   9   7   5   3   1

Library of Congress Cataloging in Publication Data

Meiburg, Albert L.
    Sound body/sound mind.

    (Potentials)
    Bibliography: p.
    1. Health—Religious aspects—Christianity. I. Title.
II. Series.
BT732.M45 1984   613   84-10356
ISBN 0-664-24532-3 (pbk.)

To the memory of
Richard K. Young
to whom the body, the mind,
and the spirit were one vital reality

and to

Wayne E. Oates
my first tutor in the art of pastoral care

gifted healers
faithful friends

Contents

Foreword

The eleven books in this series, Potentials: Guides for Productive Living, speak to your condition and mine in the life we have to live today. The books are designed to ferret out the potentials you have with which to rise above rampant social and psychological problems faced by large numbers of individuals and groups. The purpose of rising above the problems is portrayed as far more than merely your own survival, merely coping and merely "succeeding" while others fail. These books with one voice encourage you to save your own life by living with commitment to Jesus Christ, and to be a creative servant of the common good as well as your own good.

In this sense, the books are handbooks of ministry with a new emphasis: coupling your own well-being with the well-being of your neighbor. You use the tools of comfort wherewith God comforts you to be a source of strength to those around you. A conscious effort has been made by each author to keep these two dimensions of the second great commandment of our Lord Jesus Christ in harmony with each other.

The two great commandments are summarized in Luke 10:25–28: "And behold, a lawyer stood up to put him to the

test, saying, 'Teacher, what shall I do to inherit eternal life?'
He said to him, 'What is written in the law? How do you
read?' And he answered, 'You shall love the Lord your God
with all your heart, and with all your soul, and with all your
strength, and with all your mind; and your neighbor as yourself.' And he said to him, 'You have answered right; do this,
and you will live.' "

Underneath the two dimensions of neighbor and self there
is also a persistent theme: The only way you can receive such
harmony of thought and action is by the intentional re-cen-
tering of your life on the sovereignty of God and the rapid
rejection of all idols that would enslave you. The theme,
then, of this series of books is that these words of Jesus are
the master guides both to the realization of your own potentials and to productive living in the nitty-gritty of your day's
work.

The books in this series are unique, and each claims your
attention separately in several ways.

First, these books address great social issues of our day,
but they do so in terms of your own personal involvement
in and responses to the problems. For example, the general
problem of the public school system, the waste in American
consumerism, the health hazards in a lack of rest and vocational burnout, the crippling effects of a defective mental
outlook, and the incursion of Eastern mystical traditions into
Western Christian activism are all larger-than-life issues. Yet
each author translates the problem into the terms of day-to-
day living and gives concrete guidelines as to what you can
do about the problem.

Second, these books address the undercurrent of helplessness that overwhelming epidemic problems produce in you.
The authors visualize you throwing up your hands and saying, "There is nothing *anyone* can do about it." Then they

show you that this is not so, and that there are things *you* can do about it.

Third, the authors have all disciplined themselves to stay off their own soapboxes and to limit oratory about how awful the world is. They refuse to stop at gloomy diagnoses of incurable conditions. They go on to deal with your potentials for changing yourself and your world in very specific ways. They do not let you, the reader, off the hook with vague, global utterances and generalized sermons. They energize you with a sense of hope that is generated by basic information, clear decision-making, and new directions taken by you yourself.

Fourth, these books get their basic interpretations and recommendations from a careful plumbing of the depths of the power of faith in God through Jesus Christ. They are not books that leave you with the illusion that you can lift yourself and your world by pulling hard at your own bootstraps. They energize and inspire you through the hope and strength that God in Christ is making available to you through the wisdom of the Bible and the presence of the living Christ in your life. Not even this, though, is presented in a namby-pamby or trite way. You will be surprised with joy at the freshness of the applications of biblical truths which you have looked at so often that you no longer notice their meaning. You will do many "double takes" with reference to your Bible as you read these books. You will find that the Bread of Life is not too holy or too good for human nature's daily food.

In this volume, Albert Meiburg leads the way as you and I find wellness in maintaining the inseparability of the soundness of body and mind. He encourages you and me to take charge of our own life-style. Under guidance from God and through the power of the Holy Spirit, we can assure health of body and mind and lay hold of the renewed energies God releases for us when we consecrate our bodies and minds to him.

Albert Meiburg introduces you to some of the latest and most significant research on the influence of your way of life upon your wellness or lack of health. Yet he translates these findings into highly readable and understandable language. If you want to read the technical sources, you can find them listed in a rich and varied bibliography. Furthermore, Meiburg tells stories of unforgettable wisdom. He shares his own pilgrimage of wellness and his encounters with illness in himself and those near to him. The result is a very human heart-to-heart conversation with you, the reader.

WAYNE E. OATES

Louisville, Kentucky

Preface

We are living in a time of great contrasts and great contradictions in the field of human health and well-being. Medical technology continues to work miracles in repairing damage and extending useful life. At the same time, the cost of high-technology medical care raises serious questions of public policy.

More is known about the interrelatedness of the various facets of wellness than ever before. The holistic health movement promises longer, more productive lives for those who are willing to take reasonable responsibility for themselves. Yet many Americans still do not see the creative possibilities that are theirs for the seeking.

Writing this book has compelled me to make a fresh appraisal of my own health and life-style and to discover ways in which I can be a better steward of my God-given strength. As you journey with me through these pages, I hope you will be encouraged to do the same.

Ever since making my first pastoral calls in the Presbyterian Hospital, Charlotte, North Carolina, I have had a special interest in the relationship of faith and health. This came into sharper focus during eighteen years of service as a hospital chaplain at the North Carolina Baptist Hospital, the

Crozer-Chester Medical Center in Chester, Pennsylvania, and the Strong Memorial Hospital of the University of Rochester School of Medicine.

My relationships with patients and with the professional staffs of these medical centers developed in me a sense of awe and reverence for the human organism—its toughness and its fragility.

I acknowledge my gratitude to Wayne E. Oates, editor of this series, for his invitation to prepare this book and for the skillful guidance and unflagging encouragement he has given. Strong support in the development of resource material came from students in my class in Health and Salvation during the spring semester, 1984, at Southeastern Baptist Theological Seminary. I thank them, too, for their colleagueship.

Virginia McDougald, my wife and companion for thirty-four years, has, more than she knows, been a contributor to this volume. I have depended heavily upon her background in nursing, her understanding of people, and her candor in helping to clarify what I wanted to say.

A.L.M.

Wake Forest, North Carolina

SOUND BODY/
SOUND MIND

Chapter 1

Can You Tell
When You Are Well?

You and I are more conscious of our health than ever before. We are more aware of our bodily functions and are
more ready to see the doctor when things are not right. We
are eating more "health foods." We are certainly taking more
exercise. According to a recent Gallup Poll, half of us exercise on a daily basis, and 81 percent believe that being in
good health is very important, second only in importance to
having a good family life.

Newspapers, magazines, television, and even records give
abundant evidence of our burgeoning preoccupation with
physical health. *Psychology Today,* after a survey of its read-
ers' beliefs about staying well, concluded in October 1982
that the intensity with which Americans are pursuing health
resembles a social and cultural neurosis. Whether this concern is neurotic or not, it is certainly strong. Anyone who
wants a little company for early-morning stretching can find
it in one of several syndicated television programs. A visit to
your local bookshop will show whole sections devoted to
diet and exercise. A case in point is *Jane Fonda's Workout
Book,* which headed the *New York Times* bestseller list for
1982. At about the same time, Olivia Newton-John made a
hit with her record, "Let's Get Physical."

However, despite this strong interest, Americans as a whole have only a superficial knowledge of health, especially concerning its more complex issues. They are prone to become enthusiasts for the latest health fads or scares, but they seldom examine them in depth. By and large they still take a crisis approach to health care. "People labor under the fantasy that the doctor can cure anything," notes Dr. Roy W. Menninger, president of the Menninger Foundation. "Also, they depend on their doctor to be knowledgeable—and don't think they have to be themselves." (Quoted in *Family Health in an Era of Stress,* p 25; Minneapolis, General Mills Company, 1979.)

Health is not the sole responsibility of the doctor. If we are to have optimum health, we must assume the major share of responsibility. This means we must make some choices. "The greatest current potential for improving the health of the American people is to be found in what they do and don't do to and for themselves," says Dr. Victor Fuchs, noted health economist (quoted in Pelletier, p. 9).*

There is a deep streak of self-destructive behavior in our culture, which must be overcome if we are to make the most of the current wave of health enthusiasm. Among the activities and habits that seriously compromise our health are overeating, smoking, overuse of medication, reckless driving, lack of exercise, and misuse of alcohol.

On the positive side, there is much that we as individuals can do to attain fitness. We can take such steps as having medical and dental examinations, watching our diets, maintaining regular exercise, and pinpointing and alleviating the causes of stress.

In the face of the current media blitz, it is important to

*See Suggestions for Further Reading for the full reference for this and other quoted material.

clarify what is meant by health. Two common images that come to mind are someone who has rippling muscles and physical energy and someone who seldom misses work because of illness.

Notice that these images symbolize a polarity. The first, physical energy, suggests a positive picture of health, while the second, the absence of illness, suggests a negative definition of health. The tendency to think about health in bipolar terms is almost inescapable and can be discovered repeatedly in historic literature of medicine and of religion.

To a degree, medicine has traditionally defined health negatively. You go to your doctor for a routine physical checkup, and if no problems surface you are pronounced free of disease or "in good health." Jesus made use of this definition of health indirectly in his familiar saying, "Those who are well have no need of a physician, but those who are sick" (Matt. 9:12).

Somehow, illness is easier to define than health. The abnormal seems more tangible than the normal. It is hard to ignore a broken bone, a high fever, or a severe depression. These are clear signs of some kind of "dis-ease." But how do we define wellness?

One positive definition of health was offered by Philadelphia physician Jesse F. Williams: "That condition of the individual that makes possible the highest enjoyment of life, the greatest constructive work, and that shows itself in the best service to the modern world. . . . Health as a freedom from disease is a standard of mediocrity; health as a quality of life is a standard of inspiration and increasing achievement" (quoted in Pelletier, p. 16).

The Greeks symbolized the positive and negative perspectives on health in the form of two deities, Asclepius and Hygieia. Asclepius, the son of Apollo, was the first physician. He became so skilled in medicine that he was thought to restore life to the dead. His sign was a serpent twined around a staff, because the serpent could shed its skin and appear young again. This emblem has come down to us today as the symbol of the physician.

Hygieia, the daughter of Asclepius, was the goddess of health in Greek mythology. She had power to cure disease. From her name we derive our word "hygiene," which stands for practices conducive to health.

Both of these deities are appealed to in the Hippocratic oath, and the emphases they represent are still with us today.

In the first century, Juvenal summed up the ideal of positive health (which gave me the title for this book): *Mens sana in corpore sano.* "A sound mind in a sound body," said John Locke, "is a short but full description of a happy state in this world."

Ironically, the same media that urge us toward fitness also often lead us to believe that our bodies are fragile things, continually exposed to serious illness, and should be carefully watched over by health-care professionals. We are faced, therefore, with the dilemma of trying to know with some degree of assurance the danger signs of serious illness while at the same time striving toward a life-style of positive health, one that will be conducive to a long and productive life. Some years ago Dr. Walter C. Alvarez put the dilemma this way: "Many persons in this world are too fearful of disease; others are not fearful enough." Striking a balance is not easy.

There was a time, not many generations ago, when infectious disease was a danger not to be taken lightly. When our children were small, I remember pausing for a picnic lunch in the yard of a German Evangelical church in eastern Pennsylvania. While the children finished their lunch, my wife and I wandered through the cemetery. We were struck by the large number of graves of infants and small children. Then we realized that these children died in the early 1800s, before medicine had made its great advances against infectious disease. Looking at our three healthy children, we had reason to give thanks.

Today, infectious disease is more nearly under control, more people survive, but we have become subject to the so-called "diseases of civilization": heart disease, stroke, cancer, arthritis, emphysema, and depression. Such conditions are usually caused by inherited tendencies, by environmental poisons, and especially by how we live. Although medicine has made strides in managing these disorders, the cost of doing so has been enormous, and the success limited.

To control the germ-caused diseases that plagued our ancestors required substantial changes in the *outer* environment, such as the introduction of modern water and sewage treatment, pasteurization of milk, and mass inoculation programs. Changes just as drastic as those programs may be necessary in our *inner* environment to control the major health problems of our own time.

For example, it is well known that heart disease, stroke, and cancer are the major causes of death and disability in the United States. Since these occur so much more often in midlife, they are felt to be potentially preventable. However, this is much more easily said than done. Measures to avoid these conditions require individuals to modify their behavior and habits of living. It is not only difficult for many people to begin new health habits, it is even more difficult for them to continue doing something that does not have a dramatic short-term payoff.

Most of us need some reinforcement to sustain a practice

that doesn't show immediate, concrete results. We are like the man I heard about many years ago when funeral homes organized burial societies. He had joined such a plan and dutifully paid the monthly dues for two or three years. Then one day he appeared in the office and announced that he wanted to quit. When asked why, he replied, "Well, I've been payin' in here for a long time now, but I don't see no benefit!"

Our insistence on having the best care money can buy has been one factor behind the spectacular rise of what some people term "technological medicine." In this approach, there is reliance on increasingly sophisticated techniques of scientific medicine, such as bypass surgery, renal dialysis, and prosthetic joints. These miracles of modern medicine can be appreciated when they extend life and enable people to live with fulfillment. There may be a problem, however, if we consistently refuse to take any responsibility for our bodies and then expect medicine to repair the damage.

In contrast to technological medicine, a broader approach is being proposed by an "ecological" approach to health care. This concept takes seriously the finite resources available to each person as well as to our planet. Proponents of this approach urge us to reduce our dependence on sophisticated biomedical technology. They are convinced that a better way to ward off the disorders of civilization is to change our self-destructive life-styles.

If the experts themselves disagree, how can you and I know what is best? The public is understandably confused when it hears conflicting testimony from one camp or another. A case in point is the frequency of warnings about the health risks of various substances that we have been eating, drinking, or using for many years without noticeable ill effects.

Sometimes people take these warnings seriously. The elderly mother of a friend of mine suddenly declined her usual egg for breakfast. When asked why after eighty-three years of eating an egg for breakfast she was now giving them up, she explained that the doctor whom she had seen the previous day had advised it, and, she added, "Why go to the doctor if you aren't going to do what he says?"

At other times conflicting testimony by health experts leads people to throw up their hands in despair. The end result, in many cases, is to reinforce our resistance to adopting positive health practices. How often have you heard someone say in response to the latest health advice, "Well, I just read last week that what they had been recommending, they now believe causes cancer! I don't believe anybody really knows what the truth is!"

Some may see scientific medicine and holistic health care as competitive. They interpret the present scene as a revolution. I prefer to think of them as either end of a continuum. As I indicated earlier in this chapter, the two interpretations are as old as Asclepius and Hygieia.

Plato recognized these two emphases in health care. He described two classes of patients and physicians. The doctors who treated slaves, he noted, never talked with their patients. They prescribed what their experience dictated and, after "giving orders," rushed off to the next patient. The other doctors, freemen treating freemen, asked questions of patients and their friends, explained the nature of the disorder, and only then would they prescribe. Plato pictures the slave doctor ridiculing the gentleman physician. "Foolish fellow," he would say, "you are not healing the sick man but educating him; and he does not want to be made a doctor, but to get well."

A balanced perspective recognizes that we need both the

technology of modern medicine and the philosophical wisdom of holistic health care because they are each useful in different areas of need.

Most of us aren't about to give up on scientific medicine. In a 1979 survey of the attitudes of American family members toward health, 79 percent of those surveyed regarded technology as the main hope for most current health problems.

One illustration of how much we rely on technology is the degree to which Americans abuse both prescription and over-the-counter drugs. We have a feeling, often encouraged by television advertising, that there should be a pill to cure whatever ache or pain we develop.

As the son of a pharmacist, I grew up with a positive appreciation of medicine and drugs. However, my father was well aware of the human tendency to deal with pain by taking a pill. Once when a new doctor in our town complained that he wasn't getting many patients, my father told him that some of his patients had complained that they went to see this doctor but received no prescription. In their minds, no drugs meant no treatment!

Even though we love technology, we also want the assurance of a human relationship with the physician. We want to retain the benefits of science, but we also look back with some wistfulness to the time when "Doc Brown" knew us and all our family as persons.

The multiplication of medical specialties, each presiding over a limited portion of our anatomy, has not made it easy to maintain the kind of physician-patient relationship we want. During a routine visit to her obstetrician, my wife once complained about an irritating postnasal drip. "Sorry about that," the specialist said summarily. "Now, how are you doing in *my* department?"

What I am saying is that if you are looking for an indignant condemnation of traditional medicine, you won't find it here. Most such outcries are based on misinformation or distortion. Blame for the shortcomings of our present system of medical care must be shared by the patients as well as the practitioners and administrators. To a large extent, the system reflects the beliefs and values of the society within which it operates.

My years as a hospital chaplain gave me a deep appreciation for the achievements of American medicine. However, over and over I have seen patients leave the hospital after being made well, only to return because of some underlying problem in their life-style, their family, or their environment.

Physicians themselves are often frustrated when their best efforts are undone by factors over which they have no control. We are beginning to see that it is precisely these factors, not usually seen as coming within the scope of traditional medicine, which have important health consequences. While not all of them are subject to our personal control, some are. It is to these areas of our experience that this book is addressed.

I hope, as we journey together, that we can explore the main avenues to wellness. A good place to start is by taking your own personal health inventory. This is the focus of the next chapter. Later we will review the danger signals our bodies give us, how our minds and bodies work together, the ways we can cope with stress, and how we can plan a program of optimum health care that will enable us to live longer, enjoy life more, and serve God more effectively.

Chapter 2

How Well Are You?

My six-year-old car got sick the other day. I began to notice a strange feeling in the steering; it seemed soft and sluggish. The car wandered around on the road. Alarmed, I took it to a mechanic, expecting him to find severe wear in the linkage, which would mean a big repair bill. A couple of hours later the mechanic phoned to say he'd found the trouble: low air pressure in the rear tires! Naturally I was relieved, but I was also embarrassed. I could have avoided this problem by simple routine maintenance.

Similarly, good health practices can prevent the onset or delay the progress of many health problems. Unfortunately, many of us take better care of our cars than we do of ourselves. People who would not begin a long trip without making sure the crankcase was full, the battery level normal, and the tires properly inflated will skip breakfast, avoid exercise, and lose sleep.

Why? I can't answer for you, but I suspect that in my own case, the answer lies in part in my unconscious fantasy of being immune from the laws of creation. Illness and accidents "happen" to other people, which is regrettable, but somehow in his great goodness God has seen fit to bestow on *me* a kind of immunity to the slings and arrows of fortune. Rationally I deny this, but at an unconscious level I'm not so sure.

If someone offered to lengthen your life expectancy by five to seven years, wouldn't you be interested? What's the catch, you ask? There is no catch. It's a fact. Most Americans could lengthen their achievable life span.

"How is this possible?" you ask. While the details may appear complex, the basic idea is quite simple. You begin by taking stock of the health hazards to which you are exposed.

By answering a checklist of questions, you discover areas of your personal life-style which, *if changed,* can materially improve your chances of survival. The benefit to you can be expressed in years of additional life expectancy.

For example, here are seven recommended health practices. Do you:

- Sleep 7 to 8 hours a night?
- Eat breakfast?
- Eat regular meals and seldom snack?
- Maintain normal weight for your height?
- Exercise vigorously at least three times a week?
- Refrain from smoking?
- Avoid alcohol?

If you answered yes to six of these questions, you have a good chance of living 7 years (for women) to 11 years (for men) longer than if you answered yes to fewer than four, according to Lydia Ratcliff, author of *Health Hazard Appraisal* (Pamphlet No. 558, Public Affairs Committee, 351 Park Avenue South, New York, NY 10016).

This may sound farfetched, but it is based upon careful research. In the early 1960s, Dr. Lewis Robbins and Dr. Jack Hall developed a new approach and a new tool while working at the Methodist Hospital of Indiana in Indianapolis.

They called their approach "prospective medicine" and their tool the "health hazard appraisal." Many other researchers have contributed to the development of this field.

The basic idea of prospective medicine is implied in its name: It looks to the future. It seeks maximum wellness, rather than waiting for illness to occur. Better knowledge of the causes and course of diseases have made it possible to predict the future results of certain past and present facts. From information about your personal and family health history, your present life-style, and certain body chemistry measures, it is possible to discover many warning signs of certain illnesses, or "precursors." These can be reduced to a few probabilities, or "risk factors."

A disease does not usually occur overnight but instead follows a predictable course. Dr. John W. Travis, a developer, with S. E. Reichard, of health hazard appraisal, has described seven stages in the history of an illness (cited in Pelletier, p. 84):

1. *No risk.* You are not susceptible to a disease agent or have not been exposed to it.
2. *Vulnerability.* You lose immunity through heredity or increased age.
3. *Exposure.* You are exposed to the agent: for example, cigarette smoke, poison ivy oil, or herpes virus.
4. *Signs.* Your diagnostic tests, such as X-rays, are abnormal even though you feel well.
5. *Symptoms.* You feel some pain or notice some change in your body or one of its systems.
6. *Disability.* You suffer limitation of function, partial or complete, reversible or permanent.
7. *Life-threatening disease.* If untreated, your illness may lead to death.

Traditionally, medical care has been concentrated on the last four stages: signs, symptoms, disabilities, and life-threatening disease. Prospective medicine seeks to work during the earlier stages, when there is a greater chance for avoiding illness or impairment.

Looking at the stages, in the natural course of an illness shows us that we don't have to wait for signs and symptoms. In many instances a careful appraisal of our personal health history and life-style reveals factors which, if they were changed, could actually add years to our lives. How do we go about having such an appraisal? There is more to it than a "routine physical," although a physical examination may be an important part of a personal health assessment.

The Health Hazard Appraisal

A health hazard appraisal is basically a checklist used to help you discover the things you are doing (or not doing) which, if changed, would reduce your chances of developing illnesses that could cause death within the next ten years.

The first step in a health appraisal is to complete a questionnaire that provides key information about the various risks you face. In addition to your age, sex, and ethnic background, the questionnaire asks for four kinds of information (Ratcliff, p. 6):

- Family and personal health history, with special attention to certain illnesses, such as heart trouble, diabetes, and cancer
- Physical measurements, such as weight, blood pressure, and blood chemistry
- Your placement in or out of a high-risk group, as shown by recent screening—such as that for breast or cervical cancer

- Life-style factors, such as food preferences, use of alcohol and tobacco, and driving habits

Just answering these questions may call to your attention some ways in which you can improve your health. For example, a doctor who specializes in physical examinations and computer-assisted audits tells in *The Rotarian* (May 1983, p. 8) of one of his patients who was quite surprised when most of his chest pains were relieved soon after he quit drinking more than twelve cups of coffee a day.

Many of us want optimum health, but we lack either practical guidance tailored to our personal health status or sufficient motivation. A health hazard appraisal offers us specific suggestions of ways to reduce our most serious risks. There is something about the prospect of several years of additional life expectancy that is positively motivating!

When you have completed the form, the information is processed by a computer or scored by hand in order to give you a personal report that includes the following items:

- Your present age in years
- Your risk age, a figure that may be higher, the same as, or lower than your actual age, because it represents the effect of all your present health factors on your longevity over the next decade
- Your achievable age, an age given in years that represents the lower risk you can attain if you make certain changes in your physical condition and health habits
- A list of major risks to your health together with specific things you can do to reduce or eliminate the risks

For example, here in simplified form is what a computer printout on Ralph Blake, a fictional patient, might look like:

HEALTH HAZARD APPRAISAL

RALPH BLAKE, White Male, 47, Wt. 197, Ht. 67, BP 148/90,
CH 278

CHRONOLOGICAL		*Recommendations*	*Benefit*
AGE:	47 YRS	EXERCISE PROGRAM	3.7 YRS
APPRAISAL AGE:	56 YRS	QUIT SMOKING	2.4 YRS
COMPLIANCE AGE:	48 YRS	LOSE 55 POUNDS	1.3 YRS
FOR COMPARABLE AGE AND		ANNUAL PROTOSIG	.4 YRS
SEX, PATIENT RISK IS 2.2			
TIMES AVERAGE		TOTAL RISK	
		REDUCTION	7.8 YRS

(Adapted from Pelletier, p. 80)

From his profile, we learn that Ralph's actual age is 47. However, because of his physical condition and life-style, Ralph's risk age is 56. He has the same chance of dying within the next ten years as a man nine years his senior. That is the bad news. But notice, also, that there is some good news!

Under Recommendations, there are behaviors that can lower Ralph's risk age. The single most important of these is exercise. If he follows a medically supervised exercise program, he can lower his risk age by 3.7 years. If he quits smoking, he can gain another 2.4 years. If he loses 55 pounds, he can pick up 1.3 years. If Ralph makes all the changes recommended, he can achieve a risk age of 48, a total risk reduction of 7.8 years.

Sometimes, the gains in risk age are even more dramatic. In the pamphlet referred to earlier, Lydia Ratcliff tells (p. 11) of a 37-year-old black woman who was in a high-risk category because she was overweight and smoked and drank excessively. Her risk age was 50.3 years. She was advised that if she stopped drinking or reduced her intake to less than seven drinks per week and did not drink before driving, her risk age would be lowered by 11.8 years. Giving up smoking would add an additional 2 years. The sum of these and all other recommendations gave her an achievable risk age of 33.5 years.

Another high-risk individual (Ratcliff, p. 12) was an 18-year-old male whose drinking and driving habits gave him a risk age of 36, double his real age! He was told that by always wearing his seat belt and not drinking before driving he could lower his risk age to 16, two years below his actual age.

Benefits of an Appraisal

Obtaining a health hazard appraisal is a good way to take stock of your health and learn how you can improve it. A physician can use it to identify high-risk patients who may need priority attention. It can also help the physician to focus the physical examination on the major risk areas of the patient.

The benefits of this sort of health assessment are fourfold (Ratcliff, p. 24):

1. It shows us the relative amount of risk for specific poor health practices, thus making clear the consequences of our behavior.
2. It makes risky behavior concrete, enabling us to realize the potential effects on our own health.
3. It offers information about the various factors, enabling us to choose which risks we want to reduce and giving us a place to start.
4. It motivates us to make changes by indicating the payoff of reduced risk.

Specialists in prospective health have documented the usefulness of the health hazard appraisal. Dr. John Milsum of the University of British Columbia found that four out of five of his patients made changes in their health practices as a result of having an appraisal (cited in Ratcliff, p. 23). Some made as many as three changes.

Similar findings were obtained in a study done under the sponsorship of NASA at the Ames Research Center in California (ibid.). Dr. Joseph LaDou and his associates reported that 80 percent of the clients who underwent an appraisal intended to make some or all of the indicated changes. The recommended changes had the potential of reducing the group's average risk age by 5 years. A one-year follow-up showed that the group had in fact made enough changes in health practices to reduce their average risk age by 1.4 years.

The Limits of Appraisal

This all sounds very well, you may be saying to yourself, but do people always follow this good advice? After all, for a long time doctors have been telling us to lose weight, stop smoking, and get more exercise. Is a computerized printout more persuasive than a physician?

Despite their enthusiasm for this new tool, the developers are not unmindful of its limits. It is more oriented toward life-threatening illness than toward chronic conditions such as arthritis, visual impairment, and poor dental health.

An appraisal may not take into account the important relationship between risks and environmental factors such as air pollution, socioeconomic status, occupational hazards, or stress. To counteract some of these limits, authorities recommend that the appraisal be supplemented with other measures of a patient's personality, emotional status, and life situation (Pelletier, p. 86).

The basis of the health hazard appraisal approach is actuarial. Its projections are based upon statistical probability. There is no guarantee that if a particular individual follows all the recommendations, he or she will beat the odds. We all know people who violate every rule of health yet appear well, while other folks who try hard to take care of themselves have poor health. Even if your risk age is 5 years younger than your actual age, your assurance of future health is only statistical, not personal.

Proponents of the health hazard appraisal recommend that it be used as a counseling tool within the context of an ongoing health-care relationship. It is noteworthy that the studies by Dr. LaDou and Dr. Milsum, mentioned earlier, were both done within such a setting. It is preferred, when the doctor sits down with a high-risk patient to review the findings of an appraisal, that the patient's spouse be present. Making the changes in life-style that are often called for will be more likely if there is a mutual understanding and effort.

You would not expect to be cured of a tumor just because your surgeon could see it on X-ray. You would have to submit to surgery, radiation, or chemotherapy, whatever treatment was indicated. In a similar way, having only an appraisal is incomplete. It can pinpoint problem areas, but, like the X-ray examination, it is diagnostic.

Screening large numbers of the population for various health risks has been done for many years, but recently it has taken on a comprehensive expression in community "health fairs," often sponsored by area health education centers. Such measures offer good opportunities for health education as well as for early detection of illness.

If you are interested in securing a personal health hazard appraisal, begin by consulting your physician. The appraisals are more likely to be available in urban areas. Some of the major medical centers are also offering wellness clinics which include health hazard appraisals.

The smart way to approach our stewardship of God's gift of life is to learn, first of all, where we stand. A health hazard appraisal is a new way to begin that assessment process, but it is not the only way. Your personal physician can help you discover how well you are. He or she can help you learn which changes in your life-style will have the greatest pay-offs for you, not just in terms of additional years but in terms of abundant life.

Chapter 3

What Is Your Body
Telling You?

Tesshi Aoyama was a student in a summer program of clinical pastoral education which I directed. While many different church groups were represented in the class, Tesshi was our only Buddhist. He had not been in this country long, and I admired the courage he showed in struggling with English and in reaching out to patients in the hospital despite cultural differences. He learned much that summer, but he also taught me a lot.

I learned that he was the twenty-second generation of his family to inherit the priesthood. For hundreds, maybe thousands, of years, his ancestors had lived in a shrine of the Jodo Shin sect. The tradition was that care of the shrine was passed from father to eldest son. Tesshi was a younger son, so he came to America to find a different place to minister.

Shrines and temples have always been places where human beings went to hear the voice of God. In Greece, people who wanted to communicate with the gods slept in temples in hopes of receiving a message in the form of a dream. Within the Christian tradition, we understand our bodies to be temples of the Holy Spirit. What does this mean practically and personally? Does it mean, for instance, that God may speak to us through our bodies? If so, what are some of the messages we may receive and how can we become more aware of them? These are issues to which we turn in this chapter.

The Body as Temple

The central figure of our faith is One whom God sent into the world in a human body. The Gospels make it clear that though he was the Son of God, Jesus knew both the joys and the sorrows of a human. He was born a baby, grew up in a home with brothers and sisters, and learned to work. He knew the physical sensations of being hungry, thirsty, tired, sleepy, frustrated, angry, and grief-stricken. He knew, too, what it was to eat and drink, to rest and relax, to scold and bless, to meditate and pray.

Early in the Gospel of John, after Jesus cleanses the Temple, his critics ask him for a sign of his authority. Jesus replies, "Destroy this temple, and in three days I will raise it up." The Jews wonder how he can rebuild in three days what took Herod forty-six years to build. John explains: "He spake of the temple of his body" (John 2:21, KJV).

In his Corinthian letters, Paul speaks of the ultimate meaning of the body. "Know ye not that ye are the temple of God, and that the Spirit of God dwelleth in you? If any man defile the temple of God, him shall God destroy; for the temple of God is holy, which temple ye are" (I Cor. 3:16–17, KJV).

In later portions of this same letter, Paul describes the diversity within the unity of the Christian fellowship using the figure of one body with its various organs under the direction of a single unifying principle (I Cor. 12:12–26).

Still later, Paul reiterates the temple motif when he declares, "Ye are the temple of the living God; as God hath said, I will dwell in them, and walk in them; and I will be their God, and they shall be my people" (II Cor. 6:16, KJV).

Careful study has led some theologians, such as John A. T. Robinson, to conclude that the concept of the body is central to Paul's theology. It is the body of Christ on the cross that is the means of salvation. In baptism we are welcomed into his body, the church, where we share his body in the observance of Communion. Our "reasonable service" to God is to offer our bodies, "a living sacrifice" (Rom. 12:1, KJV). Finally, in the resurrection, "we shall all be changed" into the likeness of "his glorious body" (I Cor. 15:51; Phil. 3:21, KJV).

The New Testament leaves little doubt that whatever concerns our bodies has spiritual significance and ethical implications. Yet the thoroughly incarnational quality of the Christian faith has not always been realized in the church.

From earliest Christian history there have been some who emphasized the difference between body and spirit. Paul struggled with the Gnostics over this. Again, in the early church, there were those who claimed that the body of Jesus was a "spiritual body" all along, and therefore different from ours. Although this teaching, docetism, was finally rejected by the great councils of the church, it has a way of reappearing from time to time.

The assumption that matter is evil lies at the heart of all efforts to separate body and spirit. If matter is evil, obviously the body is evil. If Jesus is God, how could he occupy an evil body? He must not have really had a sinful body like ours. This is the way the reasoning goes. This, in spite of the clear word in Genesis (1:31) that God looked on all he had made and called it good!

During the Victorian era, for example, the body was something to be ashamed of and overcome. This is one reason that thinkers like Darwin and Freud aroused the ire of theologians. Darwin, Freud, and others accepted the body as essential to our humanity. Now, in the twentieth century, say Carl and Lavonne Braaten in *The Living Temple* (Harper & Row, 1976, p. 7), "theology has had to make the long trek home to the body where the faith was born in the first place."

Contemporary Christian attitudes toward the body seem to range from those which are essentially *antagonistic* to those which are essentially *accepting.* Alienation from one's body may be expressed both by neglect, ignoring its basic needs, and by overt opposition, in which exorbitant demands are made upon it (as when middle-aged people overexert). The narcissistic preoccupation of those who are never satisfied with their appearance may reflect low self-esteem. The rejected body becomes a thing—an object.

Acceptance of one's one and only body arises from the realization that not only do we *have* bodies—we *are* our bodies, from the soles of our feet to the hairs of our heads. Taking the needs of the body seriously and giving it sensible care is one expression of healthy self-regard. The accepted body becomes a subject. It is surprising, when you make an honest effort to befriend your body, what an interesting conversation can ensue.

Body Messages

Social anthropologists have shown how much our bodies can communicate about us to other people without our ever saying a word. A skilled observer can learn to read these "body messages" from our posture, eye movements, facial expressions, and gestures.

Not only do our bodies communicate to other people, they can communicate to us if we are inclined to listen. Under normal conditions our bodies take care of a number of complicated biochemical processes with no conscious effort required of us. For example, I don't have to remember to perspire when I exercise vigorously. My body has already remembered to do that for me.

In his pioneering research over fifty years ago, Dr. Walter B. Cannon documented the marvelous ability of the human body to maintain its biochemical equilibrium despite broad changes in its environment. He termed this built-in gyroscopic effect "homeostasis" and demonstrated the myriad ways in which the "wisdom of the body" makes possible higher social functioning. However, when there is a period of prolonged stress, the organism will begin to send distress signals. Our bodies speak to us in several ways: They may gain our attention through changes in our sensations, our behavior, or our energy level or through illness.

Through the *sensations of our nervous system* we become aware of a variety of maintenance needs of our bodies. Hunger indicates we are running low on fuel. Drowsiness signals the need for a rest stop. Muscle restlessness may call for exercise or stretching. Pain can be a report of damage to tissues or a warning that a battle is in progress, as when a tooth is abscessed or a throat sore.

A *change in behavior patterns* is another way the body can send a message. Feelings and attitudes that might otherwise remain unrecognized may be expressed behaviorally. One of our sons sucked his finger as a baby. He outgrew this, of course. Sometimes, however, when he was especially tired or frustrated, his finger would wander into his mouth without his being aware of it, alerting us to his fatigue.

A *fluctuation in energy level* can alert us to some aspect of our lives that needs attention. While in the navy I served as an electronics technician. Sometimes the folks at the communications center complained to us at our transmitter station out in the boondocks that they weren't getting through. Usually our response was to increase the coupling of power in the final amplifier. But sometimes this only made matters worse. Then we found, strangely enough, that if we *reduced* the power the signal got through better!

Something like this occasionally happens as we pursue important goals and objectives. We go all out on a project for a time, and then we become aware that our energy is waning. Pushing ourselves even harder may not get as good results as backing off, uncoupling for a spell, and letting our organism recover its powers.

The timing and intensity of changes in energy level can be a useful body message. Typically we get "up" for things we feel are important. A feeling of sluggishness may tell us that we resent having to do something. An unremittingly low energy level is often associated with depression.

The body messages we have been discussing thus far are like conversations among friends. But occasionally the body seems to find that its well-modulated tones are ignored. When this happens, it becomes necessary for the body to shout. *Illness or symptoms of illness* may wave us off the track for a needed repair of some aspect of our lives.

I recall how surprised I was one Saturday morning at my desk when I became aware of a hole in my visual field. I was talking on the phone and trying to make notes. I couldn't see what I was writing except by using peripheral vision. I left the office and started home, remembering to pick up some shoes that I had left to be repaired.

My feelings of concern were further intensified when I tried to tell the repairman what I wanted and found that my speech was garbled. I showed him my claim ticket, paid him, and made my way toward my car.

Before I reached the car I bumped into our pastor. He

greeted me with his usual enthusiasm. I understood him, but a thick tongue kept me from giving him a very sensible reply.

By the time I reached home I was developing a splitting headache and went to bed, where I stayed for the rest of the day. The pastor called my wife and asked if I were on some kind of drug. He knew something was awry.

The headache was bad enough, but on top of that I had to coordinate a city-wide family life institute in another state the following week. I deferred my departure, and by Monday I felt well enough to travel to my engagement.

When I returned home I consulted my doctor, who gave me a careful going over, including putting his stethoscope to my head! This was a new procedure for me, but he explained that he was listening for signs of impaired circulation. He concluded that I had experienced a spasm in the blood vessels, since my symptoms were so like those of a migraine attack.

At infrequent intervals I continued to have similar episodes. Once I arrived at a commencement service where I was to give the address. In the midst of the procession I began to have the now familiar warning signals. Somehow I stumbled through the address. I don't know how many other people knew I was in trouble, but my wife did.

Finally, after moving to another state, I went for a checkup. My new internist took note of my history and gave me some medication that might reduce the intensity of the symptoms. Then he suggested that perhaps I should try to take as good care of myself as I tried to take of the patients I served in the hospital. I felt cared for and began to be more accepting of my limits. It has been almost ten years since I had one of these attacks. My doctor had helped me read the message in my illness.

Body Befriending

When illness comes, it may be useful to ask yourself if there is some aspect of your life that needs changing. Reflection may suggest that our bodies deserve more respect as God's unique gift to us. It is not always easy to take care of our selves. We are often led to feel it is selfish. In the past, women were discouraged from developing their intellects, and men were taught to subordinate their inner feelings as they pursued career advancement (Jaffe, pp. 30–31).

Some years ago I participated in a research project in a large medical center which showed me how the body can persist in sending signals that become progressively stronger if ignored. I read the medical histories of a large number of clergymen.

One pattern appeared with some frequency. On the first visit to the clinic, the patient complained of gastrointestinal distress such as cramping and indigestion. This might be treated with antacids and tranquilizers. The complaint would continue through a second visit, and the patient would receive similar symptomatic treatment. By the patient's third or fourth visit, a stomach ulcer would be discovered, usually necessitating a period of rest. In some instances the ulcer healed but later returned, and surgery became necessary.

In these persistent cases, inquiry into the social situation of the patient often showed many stress points, some self-induced. Overwork was a way of proving one's dedication.

The enforced rest that illness brings can become a time of recovery of our total well-being, not just our body's health. My friend Robert Reeves, for many years the chaplain at Columbia-Presbyterian Medical Center in New York, has traced the kind of inner pilgrimage that has led many people to reevaluate the direction of their lives as a result of something that happened to their bodies. He found that when he asked patients what meaning they saw in their illness, they usually began by describing it as an intrusion. He called this level of awareness *dissociation,* since it implied that illness was a product of purely external events, a "bug" or an "accident."

However, as he listened further, he heard patients reach a deeper level, which he called *dysfunction.* Here, illness is perceived as within, something the patient can't do. This was followed often by the revelation of a sense of *disharmony,* which Reeves described as "a sense of disaffection or alienation, a loss of meaning or direction or integrity." (Robert Reeves, Jr., "Reading the Message of Illness," an address for the Annual Meeting of the American Protestant Hospital Association College of Chaplains, 1968.)

When given the opportunity to explore his or her feelings further, the sick person often began to take *responsibility* for the illness. Confession of guilt and its resolution may then lead to the process of *redefinition* of a way of life, in which new values are embraced and important relationships restored.

What Reeves has described is a process of internal dialogue between us and our bodies. We become friends with our bodies in the same way we become friends with other persons—by showing consideration and concern. When your friend speaks, you listen. When you speak, your friend listens. Our bodies are more than encumbrances and burdens, they are *us.* They may even be the medium through which God speaks to us for our own good, and ultimately for his glory.

Chapter 4

Can Heartbreak
Break Your Heart?

Lori took a summer job in a distant state, miles away from her parents and her boyfriend. As the summer wore on, she began to have second thoughts about the future of her relationship with the young man. Communication problems with her parents also developed. One day, without explanation, she received a letter from her mother, telling her never to call home collect again. She began having severe recurring pains in her ear. Visits to three doctors failed to explain the pain or the cause.

Lori connected her ear with the telephone and concluded that her pain symbolized her feelings of anger, fear, and confusion. She noticed that when she was extremely upset, she frequently had pain in her ear.

Was Lori's experience a coincidence? Is it really true that disturbances in our emotions can result in physiological changes? If so, how are such changes brought about? More importantly, is there any evidence to indicate that emotional satisfaction is conducive to physical well-being? These are valid questions, and they deserve to be taken seriously.

Can Bad Feelings Make You Feel Bad?

Whether illness is more a product of internal or external influences is a question that goes back to the earliest days of medicine. One approach has emphasized the discovery of the laws that govern natural processes. The other has stressed the consideration of the whole organism and its environment.

For example, in the 1890s, tuberculosis was thought to be a product of social and environmental influences. When Louis Pasteur and Robert Koch showed that it could be traced to a specific "germ," they were opposed by most doctors. How ironic, notes a leading proponent of holistic medicine, that the findings of present-day researchers about the role of psychosocial and environmental factors in infectious diseases are questioned because we now have come to accept the germ theory as conclusive (Pelletier, p. 96).

We are beginning to see that these two approaches to health, the scientific and the humanistic, are not really enemies. Each has a contribution to make in our quest for maximum wellness.

But what about our question. Can bad feelings make you feel bad? The side of medicine that has stressed the role of psychosocial factors answers yes. It has long been noted by physicians that emotional disturbance may predispose a person to illness.

James Lynch, in his book *The Broken Heart: The Medical Consequences of Loneliness,* describes how loneliness and isolation are contributing factors in death by heart disease. For example, death by heart disease in the age group from 15 to 64 is twice as high among divorced men as among married ones. Similar (but not as drastic) rates are characteristic of the differences between widowed and married women ages 15 to 64. The factors of loneliness and the loss of loved ones appear very high in the emotional/biochemical disorder of depression. Lynch says (p. 41) that "in a surprising number of cases of *premature* coronary heart disease and *premature* death, interpersonal unhappiness, the lack of love, and human loneliness seem to appear as root causes of the physical problems."

Two Johns Hopkins University researchers, Caroline B. Thomas and Karen R. Duszynski, studied more than a thousand medical students over a period of eighteen years. High blood cholesterol was discovered in more than a hundred of these students, but during the period of the study only fourteen had coronary attacks. A review of the psychological data on the students with elevated cholesterol levels showed that those who did not have attacks were individuals who tested low on measures of anxiety, tension, and depression.

By contrast, the students who later developed heart attacks scored high on these scales, "tended to suffer from insomnia, were often tired in the mornings, and generally had lower grades than did the other medical students." (Reported in *Johns Hopkins Medical Journal,* 134:251–270.) Such findings suggest that biological factors, such as high levels of cholesterol, are only partially to blame for heart disease. Emotional factors play an important role. Bad feelings can make you feel bad!

Dennis T. Jaffe is a clinical psychologist who has helped many people recover their health through a comprehensive review of the various aspects of their lives. He has noticed a striking similarity among nearly all his clients. "Almost none of them felt good about themselves, nor did they spend much time taking care of their personal needs, either physically or emotionally" (p. 112).

Situational crises can generate enough stress to make you feel bad. Charles had been an extremely healthy individual all his life. Suddenly, in his early sixties, he began developing circulatory problems. After a series of tests he was treated, but each time the treatments helped only for a short time. After about a year, his doctor asked about his plans for retirement. Charles burst into tears and began to tell how fearful he was of facing the rest of his life as a "useless shell."

At the suggestion of his physician, Charles sought counseling. He worked through his anxiety and began planning a retirement that would be productive in areas for which he had not previously had time. Within three weeks his circulation problems had abated to the point at which medical treatment could be discontinued.

Charles's story sheds light on the effect of feelings on health in several respects. It illustrates, first, how a lifelong balance of wellness can be upset by an intense emotional issue. All of us are vulnerable to such stresses from time to time.

Additionally, what happened to Charles reminds us that an alarming symptom may demand so much attention in itself that it diverts attention from other important aspects of our life situation. We want our symptoms taken seriously, and they should be. At the same time, however, if we stop at the stage of symptomatic relief we may overlook the underlying message of the body.

Finally, we learn from this episode the importance of sharing our feelings. As long as Charles kept his fears to himself, they worked away at his body.

Should we conclude that feelings are dangerous? Not in the simple sense. Feelings are an inescapable part of being human. Sometimes we are tempted to avoid the pain of bad feelings through reliance on medications. A disadvantage of this strategy is the tendency of many of these substances to reduce not only our ability to feel bad but also our ability to feel glad! Given under medical supervision, drugs can help temporarily, but they are not a long-term solution to bad feelings. Remember, the same God who gave us the ability to feel also gave us the ability to think and to act.

Sharing feelings of jealousy, anger, guilt, or depression is not easy. We are seldom proud of such emotions. If we have at least one real friend to whom we can unburden ourselves, a lot of the pressure can be alleviated. "Check" Bovender, a long-time friend with whom I have shared during times of struggle, artfully inscribed this reminder on a plaque I keep in my study. It says, *A friend is one who knows you as you are, understands where you've been, accepts who you've become, and still gently invites you to grow.*

Stress on the body seems to come mainly when we feel trapped by a role. Having to keep up a front continuously drains away the energy that would otherwise be available for creative work and the maintenance of physical well-being. In the familiar novel *Doctor Zhivago,* Boris Pasternak puts it this way (Pantheon, 1958, p. 483):

> Your health is bound to be affected if, day after day, you say the opposite of what you feel, if you grovel before what you dislike and rejoice at what brings you nothing but misfortune. Our nervous system isn't just a fiction, it's a part of our physical body, and our soul exists in space and is inside us, like the teeth in our mouth. It can't be forever violated with impunity.

The power of sin to invoke illness was well known to the psalmist. In one instance, he cries out to God, "Because of your anger, I am in great pain; my whole body is diseased because of my sins" (Ps. 38:3, TEV). Keeping his feelings to himself didn't seem to help: "I kept quiet, not saying a word. ... But my suffering only grew worse, and I was overcome with anxiety" (Ps. 39:2–3, TEV). A similar passage is found in Psalm 32, attributed to David, where, in good King James language, the text reads, "When I kept silence, my bones waxed old" (v. 3). An honest confession is good for the soul, according to conventional folk wisdom. It seems apparent that it can't hurt the body, either.

How Do Feelings Affect the Body?

Anecdotal evidence linking the mind and the body has been around for a long time, as we noted earlier. The studies of Walter B. Cannon showed that measurable changes in biochemistry could result from emotional stimulation. Later research on psychosomatic illness attempted to trace specific illnesses to specific emotions, or to identify certain personality traits that seemed to predispose individuals to certain disorders. These efforts corroborated the role of emotions in illness but left unclear how the influence of feelings was mediated.

Today, however, we have new evidence of a direct physical connection between emotions and the body through the immune system. Work in a new field with the jaw-breaking name of psychoneuroimmunology is beginning to disclose the connections between the brain (where we think and feel), the endocrine complex (hormone-producing glands under the control of the brain), and the immune system.

Research is discovering that too much of certain hormones over too long a time can disturb the balance of the immune system. Different emotions produce different hormones. Anger and fear, for example, cause the adrenal glands to secrete hormones that raise the blood pressure, increase free fatty acids in the blood, and speed up the heart rate. If this process remains activated, the person becomes more subject to high blood pressure, heart disease, stroke, and migraine headaches.

Other emotions, such as feelings of loss and failure, cause the adrenals to produce different hormones. They, in turn, can foster the so-called autoimmune diseases, including rheumatoid arthritis, lupus erythematosus, and pernicious anemia.

Laboratory studies in neuroimmunology are showing more precisely how the mind affects immunity. Psychologist Robert Ader and immunologist Nicholas Cohen of the University of Rochester have been able to "teach" rats to suppress their immune response. Dr. Ader was using behavioral conditioning methods to make rats averse to saccharin. He used a drug to give the rats an upset stomach. It worked very well. They acquired an aversion to saccharin in just one session.

Unexpectedly, after about forty days, some of the animals died. In trying to figure out why, he learned that the aversive drug not only made the rats feel bad but also suppressed their immune response. This made them more susceptible to infection.

In collaboration with Dr. Cohen he designed further experiments in which mice reacted to saccharin as if it had been the immunosuppressant drug. The mice "thought" their immune systems were working poorly, and, in fact, they were. The Ader-Cohen findings, now confirmed by other independent researchers, show that it is possible to train mice to suppress their bodies' normal resistance to foreign protein. "As recently as 10, even five years ago," Dr. Ader noted, "there were no readily accepted connections between behavior and the immune system." (Quoted by Alan Anderson in *Psychology Today,* December 1982, p. 55.)

The implications of these findings for human health are encouraging, for they suggest that individuals may be able to "learn" how to strengthen their immune response, thus rendering them more resistant to disease.

Can Good Feelings Help You Feel Good?

My wife and I were invited to a neighbor's house for dinner recently. Our host is especially gifted as a storyteller, and he was in good form. He has a droll sense of humor. I love to be around him, because I know that when I leave I will feel better than when I came. This night was no exception. For more than an hour during and after dinner we had a rollicking good time. When, after I had dried my eyes for the tenth time, we reached home, I felt completely relaxed and rejuvenated.

No doubt you have had the same sort of experience. It suggests that Norman Cousins may not be too far off base when he calls laughter "a good way to jog internally without having to go outside" (*Anatomy of an Illness,* p. 84). The words of Proverbs also come to mind: "A merry heart doeth good like a medicine: but a broken spirit drieth the bones" (17:22, KJV). I like the way the Good News Bible: Today's English Version renders this verse: "Being cheerful keeps you healthy. It is slow death to be gloomy all the time."

If psychosocial factors can create vulnerability to illness, as new research seems to show, it follows that such factors may also help in achieving wellness. Disease-fostering forces, such as genetic disposition, environmental stressors, and infectious agents, may be thought of as children lined up on one end of a seesaw. Disease-fighting forces, such as good nutrition, the ability to cope with stress, and the immune system, are arrayed on the other end. When the balance is delicate, the addition of even a small force—hope, for instance—can make a difference.

"It makes no sense to believe that only the negative emotions have an effect on the body's chemistry," declares Norman Cousins in an essay, "Healing and Belief" (*Saturday Evening Post,* April 1982, p. 48). "Every emotion, negative or positive, makes its registrations on the body's systems." Widely known as editor of the *Saturday Review,* Cousins made a remarkable recovery from a life-threatening illness almost twenty years ago. How he regained his health through a partnership with his doctor and "large doses of love, hope, faith, laughter, confidence, and the will to live," is told in his bestselling *Anatomy of an Illness.*

More recently, on December 22, 1982, Cousins suffered a heart attack. In facing this latest health challenge, he discovered that the "old" program from his previous illness was still "both accessible and working" (*The Healing Heart,* p. 53). He asks (p. 119), "Is it possible that irregularities of the heart rhythm and even problems of blood pressure should be treated not just chemically but also emotionally and spiritually? Attitudes may be just as important in repairing the heart as they are in combatting other assaults on human health." This spiritual and emotional regeneration of the heart calls for a "systematic regimen of careful diet, regular exercise, control of stress and a philosophy of life that provides ample nourishment for the generous appetite of the spirit."

In his essay "Healing and Belief" (p. 31), Cousins calls the body's ability to heal itself "the greatest force in the human body." But he also argues for the critical significance of "the belief system, which can translate expectations into physiological change. . . . Everything begins, therefore, with belief," he asserts. "What we believe is the most powerful option of all."

The reality of which Cousins speaks was confirmed by one of my students. She experienced a severe emotional trauma while serving as a church staff member. Because her husband's career was at stake too, she felt helpless to do anything to make the situation better.

She and her husband moved to a new community. Eighteen months after the traumatic incident she was diagnosed as having a probable lymphoma. Following two biopsies her hematologist recommended that she maintain care in nutrition, exercise, and life-style but defer chemotherapy for a time. She continues regular check-ins with her doctor but in two years has had only two flare-ups. She seems to be using the belief system to advantage.

We began this chapter asking "Can heartbreak break your heart?" Heartbreak and loneliness, as well as other bad feelings—anger, guilt, and helplessness—can have a negative effect on health. But the good news is that good feelings—laughter, hope, a sense of purpose, and faith—can often tip the scales in the direction of well-being.

There is great wisdom in nourishing what Cousins called "the appetite of the spirit." Heart hunger is the scriptural figure for this human need. The psalmist's heart "thirsts for God." God examines our hearts and is acquainted with our inmost thoughts. We open our hearts to God through the experience of prayer, meditation, and worship. Cultivating the spirit keeps our hearts tender (Eph. 4:32). Indeed, it is the "hardening of hearts" (Matt. 19:8) that ruptures relationships and spawns loneliness, much of which is self-chosen and is a subtle expression of the will to die rather than the will to live.

Chapter 5

Is Stress Your Friend or Your Enemy?

In 1963, Lowell Thomas, the famous world traveler and news commentator, was hospitalized with complaints of dizziness, fainting, extreme fatigue, and muscle tremors. His physicians suspected a heart attack, but the usual tests did not bear this out. It was only when the patient himself began to think about what he had been doing lately that his problem was diagnosed.

For several months, Thomas had been traveling around the world nonstop. His journeys had taken him across all twenty-four time zones. Although some of his symptoms were those of a heart attack, in reality he was suffering from severe jet lag.

When the advent of jet aircraft made it possible to travel great distances in a short time, millions of people began to suffer from this new stress. Scientists who study body rhythms have shown that jet lag occurs when we travel in an east/west (not north/south) direction too rapidly for our bodies to adjust to a new time frame. They have also discovered ways to help travelers prepare for and offset the effects of this particular stress. The methods include adjusting one's diet, rest cycle, and exposure to light, which signals the body's hormones to cooperate with the new time frame.

Jet lag is only one of the many forms of stress that we are subject to as a result of living in a technological society. Other environmental sources of stress in an urban area are noise levels, water and air pollution, population density, and traffic congestion.

The potentially hazardous effect of stress on health has been widely publicized in recent years. In a national survey of family health attitudes and behavior sponsored by General Mills in 1978–1979, 82 percent of the respondents said they needed less stress in their lives.

Despite our current preoccupation with stress, it is not a new phenomenon. Although the word itself is not found in the King James Version of the Bible, the experience is certainly there. The stress vocabulary of the Bible, Wayne Oates points out, includes such terms as affliction, distress, perplexity, tribulation, and trouble. The apostle Paul is a case in point. He wrote to his friends in Corinth describing "the affliction we experienced in Asia; for we were so utterly, unbearably crushed that we despaired of life itself" (II Cor. 1:8). Yet we think burnout is a new phenomenon! And there was more to come. "Even when we came into Macedonia," Paul continues, "our bodies had no rest but we were afflicted at every turn—fighting without and fear within" (II Cor. 7:5).

An example of a seventeenth-century stress disorder was recently reported in the *British Journal of Psychiatry* by R. J. Daly of the University College in Cork, Ireland. During the eight months following the Great Fire of London in 1666, Samuel Pepys showed repeated symptoms of psychological distress, including an obsessive fear of fire, sleep disturbances, impaired memory, and irritability.

The disastrous effects of stress first came to medical attention on the field of battle. During the Civil War, palpitations were seen so commonly that they were termed "soldier's heart." Over fifty years later, in World War I, the mental confusion of troops following long exposure to heavy artillery bursts was called "shell shock," since it was first thought to be due to damaged blood vessels in the brain. The problem was seen again during World War II, but then it was called "battle fatigue."

During the 1930s, physiologists had shown that psychological strain could produce decided shifts in the levels of certain hormones. Building on their work, Hans Selye, the father of stress research, discovered many of the biological mechanisms by which stress impacts the body. He showed that when there is no relief from a stress situation, high blood pressure, high levels of cholesterol, and depression of the immune system can result.

Selye found that the body uses the same adaptive-defensive mechanism to meet a wide variety of stress conditions. He termed this indiscriminate biological response the "general adaptive syndrome." In his own words (pp. 256–257),

> We have learned that the body possesses a complex machinery of checks and balances. These are remarkably effective in adjusting ourselves to virtually anything that can happen to us in life. But often this machinery does not work perfectly; sometimes our responses are too weak, so that they do not offer adequate protection; at other times they are too strong, so that we actually hurt ourselves by our own excessive reactions to stress.

What determines whether stress is our friend or our enemy? Is some stress beneficial? If so, in what way? How can we learn to handle the stresses we can't avoid so they don't impair our health? These are intriguing questions.

Stress as Enemy

A drawing accompanying a recent magazine article illustrates a popular conception of stress. It shows a poor soul suspended in midair with no less than seven huge hooks pulling at him from every direction. The various hooks are identified by such labels as "financial pressure," "global tension," "marital stress," and "business pressure." Emotionally, the drawing is accurate, because under stress we often *feel* pulled in many directions. Actually, however, the drawing is misleading because it portrays the stress sufferer as a helpless victim of completely external forces.

Is stress your enemy? Researchers help us at this point by distinguishing between the things that cause stress, "stressors," and our reaction to them, which is more properly called "stress." A stressor is an enemy in that it can trigger the "stress reaction," which is the way the body responds to a perception of threat.

According to Selye, the body responds to threat in three distinct stages:

1. *Alarm.* The brain sends chemical messengers to the pituitary and adrenal glands, and these glands release hormones that raise the level of blood sugar, speed up the metabolism, raise the blood pressure, and speed up the heart. We are prepared to fight or run. This is an emergency alert. It cannot be maintained indefinitely.

2. *Resistance.* After the alarm has been sounded, the body goes into overdrive, taxing its energy reserves in order to resist the focal stress. Concentration on one threat tends to lower the body's ability to resist

other hazards. Thus, preoccupation with a threat to self-esteem, for example, could result in less resistance to infection. Some illnesses, such as hay fever, seem to be caused by more resistance from the body than the outside stressor deserves.

3. *Exhaustion.* When the supply of adaptive energy is temporarily exhausted, the body is no longer able to defend itself. Muscles no longer function, or they become cramped. Mental activity slows. Sleep comes. With rest, energy is renewed.

Selye suggested that each person has a lifetime supply of adaptive energy, which can be drawn on in emergencies, like money in the bank. Unlike money, however, it cannot be accumulated, nor does it earn interest. It can only be partially replaced by rest. The cumulative deficit between the expenditure of adaptive energy and its partial replacement is what Selye called aging. The unusual longevity of residents of certain communities, such as the Italian families of Roseto, Pennsylvania, and the inhabitants of Soviet Georgia, might be due to a lower exposure to stress in the form of social change. Perhaps those people expend their adaptive energy at a slower rate.

The stress resulting from significant changes in the life pattern is well known to have a bearing on health. Dr. Adolf Meyer, dean of American psychiatry in the early part of this century, used to ask his patients the dates of their major illnesses. Then, alongside these, he noted important events and frustrations. Often he discovered that major life change was followed by illness.

More recently, in the 1940s and 1950s, another psychiatrist, Thomas Holmes, and a psychologist colleague, Richard Rahe, devised a way of measuring the stress of life changes.

They asked five thousand people to assign a stress value to various life events. From these responses, Holmes and Rahe produced the now well-known Social Readjustment Rating Scale (see Appendix).

On a scale of 1 to 100, marriage was given a point value of 50. The death of a spouse, the most severe stress, was rated 100. Other high stress events included being fired from a job (47) and divorce (73). At the low end were such items as buying a car (17) and getting a traffic ticket (11). Even welcomed changes, such as marriage, birth of a baby, job promotion, and vacation are stressful and contribute to your total life change units (LCUs).

Application of the Holmes-Rahe scale to various groups has shown that it can be used to forecast the risk of illness following a period of major stress. For example, those who scored from 150 to 200 LCUs in a twelve-month period had an illness rate during that period of 37 percent. This rate went up to more than 50 percent for those with 200 to 300 LCUs, and when total LCUs were over 300, 80 percent of the group experienced illness during that period. A study of college football players disclosed that 50 percent of those who ranked in the top third in LCU scores were disabled by injury during the season, compared to only 9 percent of those scoring in the bottom third (Jaffe, p. 79).

One of my students, Marty M. Hager, imagined giving the Holmes-Rahe scale to the Old Testament character Job. He pictured Job as having heard of one catastrophe after another. His livestock has been captured and his servants killed. Then a tornado strikes the house of one of his sons, and all seven sons and three daughters are instantly killed. Despite such severe losses, Job does not complain to God. Disregarding the property losses, at this point Job already has 10×63 LCUs or a total of 630, more than double the level at which there is an 80 percent likelihood of incurring illness. Sure enough, in the next scene Job breaks out in boils from one end to the other—his unspoken grief has suppressed his immunological defense system!

The Holmes-Rahe scale can be useful in taking a reading of your cumulative stress load, but it does have certain limits. What it can predict is the *average risk* of illness. Many individuals who score high in LCUs do not, in fact, become sick. For example, Harold J. Wershow and George Reinhart of the University of Alabama found little correlation between high LCUs and hospitalization in a study of 88 patients admitted to a veterans hospital (*Journal of Psychosomatic Research* 18:393–401). Some patients with few discernible changes in their lives became sick. The researchers concluded that further study is needed on these apparent exceptions to the rule, as well as those who seem to withstand stress well. If we knew what worked for these folks, we might be able to help others learn how to cope better.

In general, then, research shows that too much stress over too long a time can be your enemy in that it predisposes you to illness. However, this is only part of the picture.

Stress as Friend

Most of us would agree that war is one form of stress which makes everybody anxious. Recall, however, the scene in the film *Patton* when the famous World War II general, brooding over the prospect of a forthcoming tank battle, exclaims, "God, I love it!"

Stress is not intrinsically destructive. In fact, some stress may actually be beneficial. Rats are more resistant to collagen-induced arthritis, for example, when they are stressed by the attention of a cat. It is not easy to say what effect a given stressor will have on a particular individual.

Individuals perceive various stressors differently. Sanford Cohen, a Boston University psychiatrist who worked with the first astronauts, told *Time* magazine (June 6, 1983, p. 49), "I would die if I had to sit in a space capsule. [However,] John Glenn just saw it as a job and went about it in a businesslike manner."

Perhaps this explains why some people enjoy hang gliding and automobile racing. "Sky-divers get hooked on the jump," observed Dr. Paul Rosch, director of the American Institute of Stress, in the same article, and "executives arrive at the airport at the last possible minute. People today have become addicted to their own adrenaline secretion."

Because individuals do differ in their tolerance for various forms of stress, they are usually not helped by simplistic advice. In an interview in *U.S. News & World Report* (March 21, 1977, pp. 51–53), Dr. Selye suggested that a stockbroker with heart trouble should never be sent to Florida and be imprisoned on a beach for six weeks. He would do nothing but run up and down the beach and think about Wall Street. He might as well be on Wall Street and learn to accept the type of person he is and develop the disciplines that will help him live in harmony with the stress of his life.

Stress seekers may be those who thrive on a certain level or type of stress. For them, stress is the spice of life. Effective executives are often of this temperament. They thrive on the gratification of being at the center of things and of being able to get things done. While President, Gerald Ford was quoted as saying, "I can't wait to get to the office each morning to see what problems there are and try to do something about them."

Executives, however, often have a factor in their favor that not all workers do: a high degree of control over their jobs.

Industrial engineers point out that jobs which make psychological demands but give little opportunity for independent decision-making can be more stressful than those we often think of as highly pressured. People who are cooks, garment workers, and assembly-line workers have higher rates of heart disease than those who have some voice in the way they work and at what pace.

Stress can be your friend—if you like the challenge of it and if you have some degree of control over your situation. Can stress play yet another role in our lives?

Stress as Teacher

Here are some suggestions that may help you learn something from your stress. If you take a closer look at your personal stress level, you may learn something important about yourself.

Name your stress. The threat value of stress is reduced if you can move from a vague feel of irritability, fatigue, or being overwhelmed by pressure to a focus on the source of the stress. It may be due to factors in your physical environment, family relationships, work situation, health, or other personal concerns. For help in locating your stress areas, look over the list of items on the Social Readjustment Rating Scale (see Appendix).

If the value assigned to an item on this list seems too low or too high for the stress you feel, you may want to give it a different value. This inventory will give you an idea of the total amount of stress you are having as a result of events in your life. In general, the higher your score, the greater the effort you may need to stay well.

Own your stress. This calls for some meditative reflection. Consider the meaning of the events you have identified. Try to get in touch with the feelings they evoke for you. Both good and bad feelings are important. Look for that part of your stress load which you yourself are causing. Have you tried to take on too many responsibilities at one time? My faculty colleague John Carlton puts it this way. "Why is it," he asks himself, "that I always agree to do these things during my manic period, but the work always comes due during my depressed period?"

Avoid some stress. The truth is, you don't have to say yes to each and every demand that comes to you. Just because one dessert is good doesn't mean three are better. Of course there are some stresses we can't avoid. I can't decide that my father didn't die last year when in fact he did. What I can decide is what I am going to do about my grief—with whom and how I can share it. One of my friends who went through a divorce arranges to spend Christmas skiing with other friends to avoid the stress of a lonely holiday. He knows enough about that aspect of his stress to own it and to head it off beforehand.

Interrupt your stress. No one can simply walk away from *all* stress, but with a little planning you can find some ways to interrupt the routine. I remember how as a seminary student I had to spend hours daily on preparation for Greek class. Often a good friend would stick his head in my door and invite me to join him in a stroll around the nearby park. The beauty of a fall afternoon and the good humor of friendly jest brought me back to my studies refreshed.

There is great value in even a brief respite. If Jesus felt it necessary to go into a quiet place to recover his strength, how much more do we? Your quiet place may be a weekend getaway with your spouse. A new scene may give you stimulation and time to get back in touch with each other.

Occasional brief vacations are helpful, but I find that what helps me even more is some time to myself each day—to glance at the paper, catch a favorite television show, or see what is happening to the flowers and shrubs in my yard.

Enjoy your stress. Not all stress can be avoided or interrupted. Even so, a great deal of the feeling of pressure can be reduced if we can overcome the feeling of being trapped—that we have no choice. When your stress has reached its irreducible minimum, you may find it helpful to try to change the way you look at it.

The American hostages in Iran were in a pressure cooker of stress. Yet even as prisoners they discovered survival skills. Some set up their own daily routines of meaningful activities. The beautiful strategy by which one hostage achieved a sense of control was to save a bit of food from his meals. Then, when someone came into his cell, he had something to offer. He turned his cell into a living room, himself into a host, and his fellow prisoner into a guest!

The courage that enables us to endure crisis is spoken of in the New Testament as faith. In the Letter to the Hebrews, the writer addresses folks who had known the stress of imprisonment: "You shared the sufferings of prisoners, and when all your belongings were seized, you endured your loss *gladly,* because you knew that you still possessed something much better, which would last forever. Do not lose your courage. . . . We are not people who turn back and are lost. Instead, we have faith and are saved" (Heb. 10:34–35, 39, TEV; italics added). In the stressful changes of life, God may be calling us to take the next step in becoming who we were meant to be.

Stress can be an enemy, even unto death. On the other hand, it can also be a friend. But friend or enemy, it can be our teacher if we see it as a challenge to grow. What is your stress teaching you?

Chapter 6

Who Is in Charge
of Your Health?

At first he thought it was only heartburn. He had never had heartburn before, but this must be what it felt like. After all, he had just given blood the day before; surely the people there would have noticed if anything was wrong. Perhaps if he were to lie down in the truck, it would go away.

At 39, with no history of heart trouble, J. F. Hensler could not believe that the increasingly heavy pain in his chest was a heart attack. He reluctantly agreed to make a quick trip to the hospital to get it checked out, expecting to return to his woodcutting.

You have probably already guessed what the doctor told him. He had indeed had a heart attack and wouldn't be cutting any wood for a spell. Hensler's account of his thoughts and feelings during and after his heart attack (*The Rotarian,* March 1983, pp. 15–17) illustrates one of the keys to wellness: taking charge of your health.

The pain prompted a kind of conversation with himself in which he began to take stock of his situation. On the one hand, he had no history of heart trouble, family or personal, and seemed awfully young. On the other hand, he had to admit that he was overweight, smoked two and a half packs of cigarettes a day, and for eight months of the year his most strenuous exercise was getting in and out of the car.

His heart attack convinced Hensler of his need to change his life-style. He quit smoking, which he had been meaning to do for twenty years, and cut back on alcohol and caffeine. A few new cookbooks gave his wife suggestions for meals that were low in fat, salt, and sugar. He began to walk and jog an hour or so five times a week, with the enthusiastic companionship of a Labrador retriever, whose "sad brown eyes and long impatient sighs" were impossible to ignore.

Although his doctors could not guarantee Hensler that all these changes would exempt him from another attack, he is convinced that living sensibly will greatly improve his odds, and he seems to be enjoying life more than ever before. Hensler has experienced a "teachable moment." One might say he has had a "change of heart!"

Organ damage, such as that caused by a heart attack, is a rather dramatic example of a physical change through which our bodies may be telling us that we need to take charge of our health. Before the days of clock radios, there was an alarm clock that would first sound a soft alarm, followed by a louder one. It was advertised with a slogan some of us still remember: "First he whispers; then he shouts!" Subtle physical changes, such as an increase in body fat or a lowered sense of energy, may be ignored. They are the body's "whispers." A heart attack is definitely one of the "shouts."

Why wait until your body yells at you before taking charge of your health? The sooner you start running your own health affairs, the greater your likelihood of maintaining a high degree of wellness. Perhaps you should ask yourself who *is* in charge of your health, and what you can do to assume that responsibility.

Who Is in Charge Here?

You go to your doctor complaining of a pain in your abdomen. After examining you he or she asks you to come into the hospital for a CAT scan. You learn that a million-dollar machine will be taking pictures of your insides by use of computerized X-ray tomography. Divested of the clothes that symbolize your individuality, you don the anonymity of a shapeless hospital gown.

"Just lie back and take it easy," says the technician. You watch as a colorless liquid begins to drip into your veins. The technician rolls you into the next room, places you under a large metal arch, and leaves you alone, closing the door. Over the intercom come instructions: "Take a deep breath. . . . Blow it out. . . . Now hold it. . . . You can breathe now." The process is repeated, punctuated by flashes of light.

As you lie there, responding to these instructions, you think about your relationship to this machine that is photographing your insides. You just lie there while it works. Miraculously, in a matter of seconds, it knows more about you than you do.

You return home and go about your business, but you are also expecting the phone to ring. It does, and your doctor says reassuringly, "There was no sign of a tumor. Everything's fine." Your suspense relieved, you suddenly become acutely aware of your heartbeat, the familiar tick of the clock, and the joy of being alive.

It dawns on you that not only are you relieved that there is no tumor, you are also glad to be back in control. From the time you went to the hospital until the time you put down the phone, you felt a vague discomfort from having placed yourself in the hands of others: your doctor, the technician, the machine. Even though you appreciate the help of each of them, it is good to be back in charge of your life.

For a long time I assumed that good health was something over which I had little control. After all, you can't choose your ancestors. You certainly can't see any of the germs that fly about from time to time. When illness strikes (notice the implication of unpredictability), you have to consult the expert. If you do what the expert says, "take your medicine" or "submit" to surgery, you may get better. But, by and large, good health was a mystery presided over by others.

Then, one Saturday, while standing in our high school gymnasium with a hundred of my fellow townspeople, I had my own little "teachable moment." My wife and I were attending a health fair.

A question at the end of a health information checklist caught my attention. It read: "Who is responsible for your health care? _____ Your physician, _____ Your hospital, _____ Your employer, _____ Your spouse, _____ Yourself." I wanted to quibble with the checklist. After all, my doctor is the pro, right? And didn't our local hospital have all the latest equipment? And didn't my employer share the costs of my hospitalization insurance? And didn't I depend on my spouse to prepare balanced meals?

The answer to all these questions was the same: "Yes, but who is finally *responsible?*" Logic compelled me to face the truth. Standing there in the gym in reasonably good health, certainly in no immediate distress, I became acutely aware that the health-care buck stopped not on my doctor's desk but on mine.

My insight was shortly confirmed by a statement from the U.S. Surgeon General to the effect that, during a recent year, 10 percent of deaths in the United States could be attributed to biological factors, 20 percent to environmental factors, and 20 percent to inadequacies in health care, but 50 percent were the result of unhealthy behavior or life-style.

At some point in their lives, many people decide to rethink their assumptions about health. They question some of their inherited family health practices. They wonder if they need to be more proactive in the interest of health, and not just reactive to illness. You may want to ask yourself the same questions I did.

Have you ever noticed how often in the Gospel accounts Jesus involved people in their own healing? One of these, a man who had been paralyzed for thirty-eight years, was lying near the pool of Bethesda. Jesus asked him a strange question: "Do you want to get well?" (John 5:6, TEV). The man explained what seemed obvious: He had no one to help him into the healing water. Why then did Jesus ask such a question? It wasn't the only time he did so.

A similar episode occurred as Jesus was leaving Jericho en route to Jerusalem. A blind beggar, the son of Timaeus, cried out to Jesus. The crowd tried to hush him up, but he persisted. Jesus stopped and asked this blind man another strange question: "What do you want me to do for you?" (Mark 10:51, TEV).

Other instances could be cited, but these are sufficient to make the point. Wholeness does not just happen. We have to want it. We have to ask for it. We have to respond to the grace God has made available. That raises the question, How do we go about taking control of our health?

What Can You Do to Take Charge of Your Health?

There are many routes to wellness. In fact, one problem you face when you begin to take your health more seriously is that there is no authority figure who can tell you exactly what your unique needs are. There are, to be sure, many enthusiasts for this or that health fad. Don't waste your time or money on wild claims. Be suspicious of "get into shape overnight" programs, which emphasize only one aspect of fitness.

I couldn't believe a recent TV sales pitch promising that if I took a pill "not available in stores" I could lose a pound or more a night without exercise or dieting—just while I slept. It even promised that if I wasn't satisfied with the first bottle, another one would be sent free!

Now, I ask you, is that reasonable? In the first place, if I weigh myself before going to bed, and again after my morning toilet, I can measure a pound of weight loss without taking any pill at all. The problem is that my basic weight hasn't changed—it is just a fluid loss. In the second place, why should I believe that if one bottle hasn't helped, a second one will?

The Kaiser-Permanente Medical Care Program in Portland, Oregon, is famous for its emphasis on prevention. Its director of health promotion, Dr. Mark Tager, and his associate, Donald Ardell, have developed a guidebook entitled *Planning for Wellness*. In it, the authors offer a useful summary of the major ways to achieve optimal health.

The first and most basic dimension of wellness, according to Ardell and Tager, is self-responsibility. The others are stress management, environmental sensitivity, nutritional awareness, and physical fitness.

Emphasizing your responsibility for your own well-being is to your advantage. This guiding intention will help you to follow through in adopting the specific health behaviors that together will form your new life-style.

Ardell and Tager suggest a checklist of beliefs that imply a

high level of self-responsibility (p. 8). How many of these beliefs do you affirm?

- I am in control of my health; doctors, drugs, and
  medical procedures can only deal with states of illness.
- Whether sick or well, I am responsible for my state.
- The main things that affect my health are my attitudes, beliefs, and behaviors.
- If I take care of myself, I can drastically reduce the
  prospects of illness while dramatically improving my
  chances of optimal functioning.
- If I lead a wellness life-style, I can come close to my
  best potential and derive great satisfaction from doing so.

If you can say yes to these attitudes, you are already ahead
in your quest for positive health. If not, don't give up or quit.
Follow along as we discuss some other steps in the journey.
Keep asking yourself what belief will best support you in becoming the whole person God meant you to be.

Preventable illness is sometimes the penalty for not caring
or for believing that health is beyond your control. A recently published study in the *Journal of Health and Social Behavior* (24:144–146) tried to correlate people's sense of control with their health status and health behavior. Melvin and
Teresa Seeman used a scale that measured the sense of helplessness (external control) or the sense of mastery (internal
control) in their subjects. They found that those who experienced a sense of control over their own health tended to
behave in these ways:

- They practiced preventive health measures by managing their diets, exercising, and restricting alcohol
  intake.

- They tended to avoid smoking.
- They were more sensitive to the need for early detection of cancer.
- They felt better about their health status.
- They reported fewer episodes of both acute and chronic illness.
- When they were sick, they were more aggressive in their management of the illness.
- They were less dependent in their use of their doctors.

Confidence in your ability to change your health for the better is half the battle.

What are some of the next steps you can take? The remainder of this chapter suggests a process of getting from where you are in your current health to where you would like to be. Here the emphasis is on the journey rather than on how you will be traveling; several specific health behaviors are looked at in some detail in Chapter 8.

Adventuring toward your highest possible level of health involves five steps: listing your health needs, visualizing yourself at peak performance, surveying your resources, setting your health goals, and creating a personal health improvement plan.

Begin by listing your health needs. You may want to look back at the health hazard information in Chapter 2 or at a comparable assessment checklist. Of course, you will want to note any chronic conditions of which you are aware. For example, if your doctor is maintaining you on medication for high blood pressure, how long has it been since you were re-evaluated? Or, if you wear glasses, how long has it been since you had your eyesight tested?

However, you also want to go beyond the illness end of

the health continuum. Ask yourself if you are satisfied with your overall energy level.. Recall the key areas of diet, fitness, environment, and stress. These may suggest current needs.

Write down a list of ten things that are preventing you from enjoying optimal health. Be concrete and include more than just the biological measures. Your list might look something like this:

My Health Needs
1. Have my eyes checked for glaucoma and my glasses for proper correction.
2. Schedule dental examination.
3. Have blood checked for triglyceride and cholesterol levels.
4. Find more time for fun with friends.
5. Learn to manage paperwork so I don't feel so pressured.
6. Reduce weight.
7. Find more time for working in the yard.
8. Strengthen upper body and back muscles.
9. Exercise with greater regularity.
10. Improve driving safety habits. Fasten seat belt.

Once your list is made, look at it more closely. Don't let the length of your list discourage you. Notice which items may take only a minor amount of work and which may call for a long process. Take note, too, of those needs which, if corrected, will do the most for your health. Which items will you gain the most satisfaction from improving?

The next step is to *visualize yourself in peak condition.* This is the positive side of listing your needs. Take some time by yourself in a quiet spot so you can relax and begin to think creatively—even to fantasize a bit.

Recall a time in your life when you were in your most vigorous condition. Call up in your mind the sensations of being energetic, alive, and capable. Enjoy the pleasure of being
in touch with the person you can be at your best.

Hold before you this positive guiding image of your own
unique wellness. Return to it often as a reminder that the
same God who made you offers you strength from within.

A third stage in the health odyssey is to *survey your resources.* You are not alone in your quest for wellness. Think
of your family members, especially your spouse (if you are
married), as well as friends, colleagues, your church, clubs to
which you belong, and community agencies.

Your close friends can do a lot to encourage or discourage
your efforts toward maximum health. You will want to bear
this in mind as you make further plans. There may be specialized health support groups, such as Weight Watchers,
whose help is also valuable. We will take a closer look at the
social context of wellness in Chapter 7, but for now a
thoughtful review of all the possible resources may reveal
that you have many previously unclaimed allies.

Now you are ready for the critical fourth step of the journey: *set your health goals.* Look back over the list of health
needs you made in step one. How can you translate these
varied needs into clear, challenging goals? To make your
goal-setting well rounded, consider some of these areas: diet,
recreation, vocational satisfaction, stress management, physical fitness, social relationships, family life, emotional health,
and spiritual well-being.

Revising your life-style requires you to set specific, realistic, and attainable goals that can be measured and that have
an appropriate time frame. Commit your goals to writing. Instead of "reduce weight," write "I will lose ten pounds by
June 1." Keep a simple record of your progress. For ex-

ample, for a weight-loss goal, you could record your weight weekly. I find it helpful to note in my appointment book how long I jog and how far.

The final step in taking charge of your health is to use your goal statements as you *make your personal health-improvement plan.* This, again, will be more helpful if it is in written form. It need not be elaborate. Some people find it helpful to list under each goal the things they plan to do to make reaching the goal possible.

For instance, suppose I want to strengthen my relationship with my children. My goal might read "I will spend six hours each week with my children during this school year." In implementing this goal, it is helpful to spell out some of the activities this calls for.

- I will spend thirty minutes a night reading to and with the children at bedtime.
- I will arrange to spend a part of Saturday with each individual child in an activity we agree on together.
- I will plan one special outing with the children each month.

Arrange your plan so that you can begin to work on some goals immediately. Pace yourself, however. It is better to have some early success, even if your goals are modest, than it is to try to do too much too fast. Bear in mind that it takes several months for new behaviors to become habits. Set some intermediate goals. They provide encouragement along the way. For more detailed guidance, consult Ardell and Tager's *Planning for Wellness.* Your greatest payoff will be the excitement of becoming more nearly the person God intended you to be.

One final word. Taking charge of your health is your right and privilege. I believe this, and I am trying to live by it myself. However, I do not mean to convey that if we follow all the health rules, we can avoid all illness. Health comes by bringing into dynamic balance many aspects of living. Doing all the "right things" for health can become a form of legalism.

Paul reminded us that we could keep all the laws, but if we lacked love we were worth nothing. Don't let your pursuit of wellness turn you into a slave, a drudge, or a crank. Health may be more a matter of living in grace than it is the result of our own efforts to keep the law. Grace to you!

Chapter 7

Who Is on Your Health-Care Team?

"Premature senility" was what the psychologist at the vocational rehabilitation service had told my 50-year-old sister, Pat, after completing a psychological examination. When she first repeated this to me, I was as puzzled by it as she was. I urged her to see a medical doctor and have a thorough physical examination.

Apparently she had been having some trouble keeping on top of her work in the state department of public welfare. Visits to her doctor and to a neurologist brought a diagnosis of Alzheimer's disease, which still meant nothing to me until Pat's supervisor met with us on a Saturday morning. He understood what we were facing. He explained that this was a brain disorder, the cause of which was unknown and for which there was as yet no cure. His mother had been given a similar diagnosis several years earlier and was now in a nursing home.

Pat had been a widow for twelve years and had no children. She lived by herself. Only a few months earlier she had sold her house and bought another. It was an attractive, modest little place, but she loved and enjoyed it. As we began to prepare for what was to come, her friends made it clear they wanted to help her stay in her own home as long as possible.

Since I lived five hours away, I kept in touch by phone and made occasional visits to see how things were going. When she could no longer drive, one of the secretaries arranged to pick her up and bring her home from work. She also arranged Saturday trips to the hairdresser. When she began having trouble with her checkbook, another friend would come over each month and write the checks for her bills.

Eventually, of course, her disability resulted in a medical retirement. Unfazed, her friends stepped up their help. To every loss, they seemed to find a compensation. Noticing a weight gain, one of them took her along to Weight Watchers. When she could no longer fix meals, a friend engaged Meals on Wheels. When she lost the ability to dial the phone, a friend had a one-button dialer installed. When she began having trouble dressing, a friend helped us find a part-time companion. Finally, it was one of her friends who alerted us that the time was near for full-time care.

Pat could never have spent that last year in her own home without the aid and support of her friends. They became family, helping in dozens of practical ways but, more importantly, sharing her frustration, confusion, and despair. They could not alter the inexorable progress of the disease, but they kept her in touch with her identity and buoyed her morale by provoking her innate sense of humor.

Perhaps you (or someone you love) have lived through a personal crisis sustained by a loving family, faithful friends, or a caring church. If so, you are already aware of the central issue of this chapter: In what ways is our health influenced by our relationship to significant others? Put in more practical terms, how can we discover and maintain a support system that will defend us against illness and enhance our well-being?

"We-ness" and Wellness

Is there any evidence that the connection between "we-ness" and wellness is more than a mystical one? Anthropology, sociology, and psychology point to the fact that throughout history human survival has depended upon interdependence.

Social obligation, says Robert Ardrey, was born on the African savanna. A prehuman hunting band of nine to eleven males supported a society of about fifty. Unfortunately, nature did not design our ancestors for hunting. They lacked power, speed, and weapons for killing. Since they did not yet have bow and arrow, killing had to be done at close range—a hazardous operation at best.

Ardrey visualizes this little band, led by a wily leader, slowly and silently circling its prey, in a fashion not unlike that of a wolf pack. They faced danger together. As he puts it (p. 329), "In trust we lived; in trust we died. And the social integrity of our little group was our one assurance of survival."

A sense of social solidarity marks the stories of Israel's conquest of Canaan in the Old Testament. The classic example is that of the sin of Achan (Joshua 7). Joshua, dismayed at the failure of the attack on Ai, asks God why. He learns that Israel has broken its covenant whereby the spoils of war were to be devoted to the Lord. Achan confesses that he has the contraband. Consequently, not only is he stoned but his sons and daughters, his herds, his tent, and all he has are destroyed. The penalty seems drastic to us because of our individualistic bias, but it also shows the importance of covenant in that day.

The New Testament church, as we see it in the book of

Acts, was a healing, life-sustaining, and sharing fellowship: "The company of those who believed were of one heart and soul, and no one said that any of the things which he possessed was his own, but they had everything in common" (Acts 4:32). Here, again, a break in the integrity of the community occurred in the sin of Ananias and Sapphira. Peter made it clear that the issue was not the partial gift of Ananias. What struck at the life of the church was Ananias' dishonesty. There can be no real community without trust.

Suicide may be the ultimate result of the loss of "we-ness." The French sociologist Emile Durkheim, in a pioneer study of this phenomenon around the turn of the century, found that the rate of suicide was greatest among people who lived isolated lives or whose cultures offered less guidance and closeness (Jaffe, p. 131). In Durkheim's setting, this meant urban, Protestant, widowed, and divorced people. Lower rates of suicide were found among the rural, Catholic, and married population.

How healthy a rural environment is may vary, to an extent, with how rural it is. The homesteaders of the American West often had more isolation than they needed. The first "little houses on the prairie" were typically built in the middle of a quarter section (160 acres), so the new owners could feel that all the land they saw belonged to them.

This isolation, says Bruce Larson, did "strange things to people" (p. 60). The actual photographs of these pioneers bear little resemblance to how we see them on television: "Weird men, wild-eyed women, and haunted-looking children" stare back at us. Before long, the settlers moved their houses to one corner of their land, where they could be close to three other families. Together they could help one another in their struggle to make a new life.

Larson's comment reminded me of how puzzled I was as I

first rode through France on the train. I saw broad cultivated fields but few farmhouses. Then I learned that since feudal times the peasants had lived in villages under the protection of the lord, close to the church and to one another.

The social values of a given community have a direct impact on the health of its inhabitants. For example, Dennis Jaffe compared health statistics of Utah with those of Nevada. Utah's population is 72 percent Mormon. Family ties and community obligation are stressed in Mormonism. Nevada's population is highly mobile, and its chief industry is gambling. Jaffe found that Utah has the lowest rate of infectious diseases, infant mortality, hypertension, cardiovascular and renal diseases, and psychological disorders of any of the fifty states. By contrast, Nevada is "at or near the top of the list in most of these same ailments." Jaffe concludes that "the social cohesion and community stability of the Mormons surely support their well-being" (p. 131).

"We-ness" as found in family ties and friendships makes for longevity, according to the research of Lisa F. Berkman, Yale University epidemiologist, and Lester Breslow, former director of health for California (*Health and Ways of Living*, Oxford University Press, 1983). Their conclusions came from an ongoing study of 4,725 men and women aged 30 to 69 in Alameda County, California. Questionnaires were completed by the subjects in 1965 and again in 1974. Ove⁻ this nine-year period, 371 had died.

The association of health practices and social networks with mortality rates was the focus of this study. As expected, Berkman and Breslow found that people practicing several high-risk habits, such as smoking, had a death rate two to three times that of people who followed low-risk practices. On the positive side, they discovered that being married, staying in touch with friends, or belonging to a church or other group may prevent premature death. The most socially isolated people in the study were more than twice as likely to die prematurely as those who had the most social contact.

The findings of Berkman and Breslow are recent confirmations of earlier studies with the same message. In the second chapter of *The Broken Heart*, James J. Lynch recounts a number of such previous studies. The thesis of his book is simple: that "loneliness and isolation can literally 'break your heart' " (p. 8). The remedy: "Quite literally, we must either learn to live together or face the possibility of prematurely dying alone" (p. 4).

If "we-ness" is so powerful, why not use it in therapy? That was the conclusion of psychiatrist Ross V. Speck, who developed the idea of network intervention while working with families with a schizophrenic member. In about 20 percent of his cases, he noticed that treating only the patient and the patient's family was ineffective.

Network intervention is simple in its basic outline but requires skillful direction. After explaining the process to the family, the therapist asks them to make a list of relatives, friends, co-workers, and neighbors totaling at least forty people. The family then becomes responsible for calling these people and explaining that they have a family emergency. Friends are asked to come to the family's house for two meetings, two weeks apart, to help them work out their problems. At this stage, the goal is to reestablish support by contacting and confiding in friends and relatives.

When those forty people have assembled, the therapist explains the purpose of the meeting, perhaps leads in a warm-up exercise, and invites the participants to reveal any secrets they know about the family! The first session frequently moves toward a polarization phase, with participants choosing up sides. Family members are invited to name several people from whom they want help. A dozen or more "activists" are organized into committees to help accomplish concrete goals, such as finding one member a job or giving another some daily attention.

At the second meeting, the activists report on what they have been able to accomplish. Usually some goals have been achieved, but not all. The family is encouraged to share their feelings and to tell the group what they want from the network. The second meeting may end with dual feelings of elation and exhaustion as support committees meet to plan further efforts. These key friends may meet sporadically for several months.

My purpose in describing this imaginative intervention is to illustrate the strength that is still available in social networks. Its innovators say that in crises where nothing else has worked, network intervention provides "the one thing that people in trouble need—a feeling that they are loved and cared about by a group of people who will support them in the future." (Quoted by Jody Gaylin in *Psychology Today,* March 1977, p. 122.) Moreover, benefits are not limited to the ill person, but are also experienced by all participants, a phenomenon familiar to members of various self-help groups.

Friendship and Fitness

Sports rooms and health clubs are a rapidly growing service industry. Current changes in their operating style, however, suggest that they too are taking into account that there is more to fitness than sweat and strain. The new factor being built into fitness center operations is friendship.

Dr. Judith Singer, a health consultant, suggests that fitness centers are replacing singles bars in a lot of ways: "Health clubs are great ways of making your business contacts, doing your networking and improving your physical and social life in a healthy environment" (quoted in *Sky* Magazine, April 1983, p. 34). Centers that once consisted of exercise rooms and showers now provide "full-service facilities," including restaurants, classes, meeting rooms, and day-care services. Apparently the friendship-fitness connection is one that makes good business sense.

Another expression of wellness and "we-ness" is the self-help movement. Mutual aid groups have been developing to meet specialized needs ever since the founding of Alcoholics Anonymous almost fifty years ago. Right in your own hometown you may have a group of undiscovered friends who share your particular health concerns.

For example, here are some situations for which a self-help group might be useful: For two years, Peggy and Bruce have been caring for their young child, who has cancer. They have good professional support and faithful friends, but they still feel alone in their grief. Candlelighters is a peer-support group for parents of children with cancer.

Daniel has tried medical help, diets, and pills but sees himself as a hopeless victim of obesity. If he is a compulsive overeater, he might be helped by Overeaters Anonymous.

George is dismayed and ashamed by what is happening to his wife. She is forgetful, misplaces things, and gets up at all hours of the night. The doctor says it is probably senile dementia of the Alzheimer type. George is trying to take care of her at home by himself, but he has started to have chest pains. He might benefit by participating in a family support group of the Alzheimer's Disease and Related Disorders Association.

To illustrate the extent and variety of mutual-aid groups, a directory of groups in the Chicago area alone lists nearly 700, addressing 150 types of concerns. Participation in such groups usually costs very little. Most are self-supporting and are run by volunteers. They do not supplant professional help, but they provide important links to services and usually have good ties with the local professional community. Many give significant support to family and friends of the afflicted, reducing isolation and the sense of helplessness.

Many local self-help groups are related to national networks. For information about mutual aid on a particular concern you can write to the National Self-Help Clearinghouse, 33 West 42nd Street, New York, New York 10036; (212) 840-7606. One location where research on self-help goes on and where additional information may be available is the Self-Help Center, 1600 Dodge Avenue, Suite S-122, Evanston, Illinois 60201.

In addition to self-help groups, another place where the connection between "we-ness" and wellness may be experienced is in the local church congregation. Gerald Caplan, Harvard psychiatrist, says that, next to families, religious institutions are the most universal of all groups providing support.

Candor compels us to admit that the vast health-support potential of congregations is not yet being fully realized. While many churches are sensitive to the needs of individuals and families at the point of illness, few envision fostering wellness as a ministry.

Nevertheless, when it is true to its mission, the church nourishes wholeness in a profoundly important way—as a fellowship which invites persons to discover or to renew the ties that bind them to God, to one another, and to their true selves. Faithfulness to the gospel produces a climate in which persons are respected, accepted, and loved as bearing the image of God. Repentance and forgiveness overcome the isolation of sin and guilt. Healing "from within" supports physical and mental well-being.

Churches could extend their wellness ministry in a more explicit way by sponsoring or promoting such activities as health fairs, exercise classes, or various forms of self-help groups. Programming for the special needs of such groups as singles and widowed persons is a welcome step in this direction.

The Health and Human Services Project of the General Baptist State Convention of North Carolina is a good example of how the church at the judicatory level can promote wellness. Begun in 1981, the project's purpose is to reduce health risks related to dietary habits, overweight, smoking, stress, and high blood pressure.

This mostly black church body has the potential to reach groups with high-risk factors. Blacks are three times more likely than whites to have hypertension and twice as likely to have diabetes. The key strategy is to equip church leaders to educate their fellow church members in preventive measures. They are also taught how to establish links with health departments, hospitals, and rural health centers.

The promise of this program was affirmed recently when it received a grant of $650,000 from the W. K. Kellogg Foundation of Battle Creek, Michigan. The grant will make possible the extension of the project from its original ten-county area to the entire state. Helping the 400,000 members of 1,700 churches to help themselves to better health is an exciting concept.

Forming Your Health-Care Team

How can you go about putting together a health-care team of your own? Here are some steps to consider.

1. *Make a list of friends and relatives* with whom you would feel comfortable in sharing your wellness goals. Network specialists suggest that this might number from seven to twelve. If you come up with only one or two, you may be under-networked! You might want to think of ways to increase your friendship circle, such as cultivating some folks who are now just casual acquaintances. However, the number is not all-important. One or two really close friends can offset loneliness and support your health planning.

2. *Consider joining a self-help group* if you or a member of your family has a special health concern. You may find new friends here with whom you have an instant affinity. If you can't locate a group in your locale, maybe you can help to start one.

3. *Find a partner who shares your health aspirations.* This may be someone who has gone through a particular operation you are facing, a friend with whom you plan to exercise on a regular basis, or simply someone with whom you feel compatible.

4. *Explore the resources of your church.* Participate in a small group, such as a Sunday school class. This will give you a circle of friends where you can know and be known at a more intimate level than is possible in the large congregation. And a minister who knows of your special health concerns may be able to suggest other people who share them.

5. *Use your physician as your professional health adviser.* Seek the doctor's counsel in planning goals for wellness that are within reason, arrange periodic screenings at appropriate

intervals, and express thanks for his special role in keeping you well!

Forming your own health-care team may be among the most important steps you can take toward wellness. If you have some misgivings about asking the help of others, as I often do, remember that our Creator said, "It is not good that the man should be alone." It is hard to be whole without having at least a few people around us who love us for ourselves and to whom we are committed in a relationship of trust. Remember, too, the words of the Great Physician: "Where two or three come together in my name, I am there with them" (Matt. 18:20, TEV).

Chapter 8

Can You Buy Health for Tomorrow?

Dr. Miller's patient stayed on the telephone most of the day. His body was in the hospital, but his mind was obviously on his business.

"Hey, Doc," he kidded, "why don't you get out of medicine and into a field where you can make some real money?"

"What do you mean?" asked the doctor.

"Well, I just made ten thousand bucks this morning sitting up here in bed. *Now* don't you think you're in the wrong field?"

For more than a week, Dr. Miller had been trying to get George Blanton's blood sugar stabilized within normal limits. Every day when he came by on rounds it was the same story. George kept riding him about being in the wrong field. Finally he lost his cool and let George have it straight.

"George," he said, "why don't you take the ten thousand you made this morning and buy yourself a normal blood sugar, and then we'd both be a lot happier!"

What about it? Can you buy health? Obviously you can't order a normal blood sugar over the telephone, even if you have a gold-plated credit card. Money is not the real answer to personal health.

Actually, the relationship between financial well-being and

physical well-being is rather complex. By most standards, health is proportional to economic means. For example, about 30 percent of people over 65 take vitamins to supplement their diets. Unfortunately, the poorer elderly, whose diets often lack essential nutrients, are seldom among those taking vitamins.

Purchasing power can buy medical care, but it cannot assure personal responsibility for well-being. As we have seen, the most significant way to improve health is not by constructing more sophisticated technological repair shops but by devising a life-style that leads to maximum wellness.

There is a "bottom line" cost for wellness tomorrow, but it is not just a dollar cost. The cost is mostly one of desire and discipline. How much do we want it, and how hard are we willing to work for it?

What are your prospects for health? Are you aware of particular health concerns you need to monitor, such as blood pressure or a family tendency toward diabetes? What can you do to live longer, happier, and more effectively? That is the focal issue of this chapter.

Why Just Survive? Plan to Thrive!

A decade ago, Dr. Robert N. Butler, a psychiatrist and gerontologist, surveyed the prospects facing older people in America and summed up his findings in a Pulitzer Prize–winning book called *Why Survive?* His title sums up the question some people ask when they contemplate their later years. The dread of poor health, the threat of dependency, and the specter of mental incapacity darken the threshold of the future for many.

Many of the "myths of aging" that Dr. Butler sought to correct are being discovered for what they are, cultural half-truths. In fact, recent research seriously questions the notion that the years after 60 are a time of inexorable physical decline. Here are some recent findings:

- Since the late 1960s, the death rate from heart disease among Americans over 65 has been dropping by about 2 percent a year.
- The death rate from stroke has been declining even faster—by about 3 to 5 percent a year.
- People over 80 are proportionally the fastest-growing subgroup in our country.

Not only are more people living longer, they are enjoying life more as a result of better health care. Dr. Lawrence G. Branch of the Harvard Medical School, together with Dr. Alan M. Jette, studied disability among older persons who took part in the Framingham Heart Study. "Substantial physical ability" is what he found among this fairly representative group of older Americans. Particularly exciting are his findings about the capabilities of those in the age group 75 to 84. Although they are somewhat more likely to need assistance, of this group:

- More than 90 percent are fully independent in the activities of daily living: grooming, dressing, eating, and moving about the house
- 85 percent can climb stairs
- 77 percent are able to walk a half mile or more
- 50 percent can perform heavy housework

The good health of these older people, to a great extent, results from the care they are taking of themselves. Branch says, "I suspect that the cumulative effects of changed lifestyles—quitting smoking, and better attention to diet and exercise—are now having their effects on reduced death rates from heart disease. This is probably going to contribute to yet another jump in life expectancy." (Cited by Michael Briley in "Over 80—And Doing Fine," *Modern Maturity,* Oct.–Nov. 1983, pp. 96–97.)

Another Harvard researcher, Alexander Leaf, has traveled the world to examine certain ethnic groups whose members not only live to great age but who apparently thrive while doing so. His findings show that the vision of optimal health throughout extended life is not an idle dream but a realistic possibility.

What can we learn from Leaf's study of villagers in such exotic locations as Ecuador, West Pakistan, and the Soviet Caucasus? Despite wide variations in elevation and climate, the settings all offered an environment of high quality. Characteristics that Leaf found common to these communities of centenarians offer several clues to wellness and longevity.

One factor of significance is the continued involvement of elders in family and community affairs. They remain active in the chores of farming and natural labor. There is no retirement. In Ecuador, for example, Leaf found no idle old people and none living alone. As they approach the age of 100 they are termed *los viejos,* "the old ones," indicating their increased social status, and they may be called on for such roles as presiding over community councils.

A second factor that contributes to wellness and longevity is nutrition. The people in these communities eat mostly vegetables, whole-grain breads, low-fat cheese, and buttermilk, but very little animal protein—less than 2 percent of their total diet. They also use only about one third the amount of fat we do. Their total daily caloric intake is about two thirds that of the average American: 1,700 to 1,900 as compared to 3,300 calories. Although the diets in these communities of centenarians do not conform to nutritional standards commonly used in this country, Leaf found virtually no one who was either malnourished or obese (Pelletier, pp. 191–203).

The third and most important factor associated with good health and long life in the villagers studied by Leaf is physical activity. In order to farm the rugged hillsides of these communities, the inhabitants have to do a lot of walking and climbing. After carefully examining the people of the Caucasian villages, Leaf found no evidence of osteoporosis and concluded that regular lifelong exercise protected the inhabitants against both this ailment, common to Americans, and heart disease as well.

Leaf's conclusions are confirmed by the findings of longitudinal studies in the United States. Not only is it possible to live into the ninth or tenth decade of life, it is possible to thrive. So if you are wondering about how to maintain your health into your later years, take heart. Why think just in terms of survival? Plan to thrive!

Why Take Chances? Make Choices!

It may seem like a digression here, but indulge me. Read the following definition of illness and decide whether you agree or not: "an entirely unwanted, useless, purposeless misfortune, acquired inadvertently through an unfortunate concatenation of forces . . . or from the defective architecture of a hereditary constitution."

What do you think? If you laughed, were amused, or shook your head, you are in good company. The quotation is from an address given by Dr. Karl Menninger, the Topeka psychiatrist, to the American College of Physicians, entitled "Changing Concepts of Disease." In the address, Dr. Menninger was confessing what he believed about illness when he graduated from medical school: the sick person was "struck down by a cruel blow from an unheeding Nature—an infestation, a lurking bacterium, a malignant cell."

Of course, he went on to show how the simplistic model of academic medicine he had learned in school did not fit the realities of the patients who came to him. He learned by experience that illness is not just a matter of chance. "It is *of* the patient, and largely his own doing." (Bernard H. Hall, ed., *A Psychiatrist's World: The Selected Papers of Karl Menninger, M.D.,* p. 671; Viking Press, 1959.)

If the holistic health movement has taught us anything, it is that we don't have to be the victims of chance nearly so much as we once thought. While it is true that we have limits, it is also true that we have a significant degree of freedom. So why take chances with your future health when you can greatly improve your odds by making important choices?

Here is a list of certain key areas of choice, with a few points under each to help you get a more concrete idea of how you can shape your health today and tomorrow. Reviewing this list may give you concrete ideas for drawing up your own wellness plan, as described in Chapter 6.

What's for Dinner?

You may think it odd, but I enjoy an occasional trip to the supermarket. I remember the excitement of the first food forays my wife and I made as newlyweds. Our budget was slender, which made shopping a kind of challenge. Along with the necessary staples we tried to find one special delight—fresh strawberries were one of her favorites and dessert figs were mine.

Whether you hate grocery shopping or enjoy it, the supermarket symbolizes the nutritional choices that can have a significant effect on present and future health. Only a day or so ago, I stood in the checkout line and watched a man in front of me. It wasn't a fair assessment of his diet, I'm sure, but I couldn't help noticing that he had only three things in his basket: a pound of lard, a six-pack of beer, and a carton of cigarettes—all the necessities of death!

Yet in spite of the tremendous number of options that a food store offers us, most of us are creatures of habit. We formed many of our eating habits early in life. Food preferences, our likes and dislikes, are notoriously resistant to change. For most of us, food is endowed with meaning, and for some of us it is overendowed.

You can start a conversation almost anywhere anytime these days by using one word, diet. Like fitness, nutrition has the capability of assuming the role of a fad if it is not approached with some basic information, reason, and balance.

One basic choice you face in the nutrition area is *what* to eat. A simple, general guide, *Better Health in Later Years* (Public Affairs Pamphlet No. 446), suggests that your daily diet should include the following elements:

- Milk, low fat, or its equivalent (cheese, ice milk, yogurt, cottage cheese)—two or more cups a day
- Protein—at least one serving daily of poultry, fish, or meat (dry beans, peas, and nuts are substitutes); one to four eggs a week
- Grain products (cereals, rice, noodles, macaroni, bread)—four or more servings daily
- Fruits and vegetables—a minimum of four servings a day; for vitamin C, at least one serving of citrus fruits and tomatoes (dark green and deep-yellow vegetables are rich in vitamin A)
- Fats (margarine, butter, salad oils, shortening, or mayonnaise)—three pats or teaspoons daily

Of course, this guide is a general one. If you have a health problem, you should adapt your diet in keeping with your doctor's advice.

Nutritionists today are recommending that we cut back on red meat and restrict our intake of salt and refined sugar. Remember that regular balanced meals of moderate size with no snacking in between was one of the health habits Lester Breslow of UCLA found to be associated with better health and longevity. Another was starting the day with a good breakfast.

A second basic choice concerning diet is *how much* you eat. As we noted earlier, communities of centenarians seem to do well on 1,700 to 1,900 calories per day. This is within the range recommended for women at age 65. For men, the figure should be no more than 2,400 to 2,600. We require the same nutrients throughout life, but as we grow older we need fewer calories. Obviously, the energy requirements for individuals will vary because of varying degrees of activity.

If you have particular concerns in the nutritional area, consult your doctor. In some communities, personal nutritional counseling is available from registered dietitians (R.D.s) qualified by the American Dietetic Association.

However, don't let the issue of nutrition get out of perspective. Food is not primarily for therapy but for enjoyment. One choice you can make is to take the time to enjoy it!

Why Run When You Can Walk?

Another area of choice that affects longevity and health is exercise. When the urge to exercise hits some people, they lie down until it goes away. That is one choice. However, increasing numbers of Americans are making another one. A survey several years ago found that 36 percent of Americans exercise regularly. Probably the proportion is even higher today.

Different forms of exercise provide various benefits. Some, such as stretching routines, improve body tone and flexibility. Other exercises, such as weight training, build strength. A third form of exercise is endurance or aerobic activities, which improve the functioning of the lungs, the heart, and the blood vessels.

Aerobic exercises include running, jogging, swimming, and biking. For you to derive real benefit, the exercise must elevate the heart rate for a sustained period of time, such as twenty minutes, and be practiced four to six times weekly.

Perhaps the best-known authority on aerobic exercise is Kenneth H. Cooper, a Canadian physician who now directs the Aerobics Center, a research facility, exercise center, and medical clinic in Dallas, Texas. Dr. Cooper discovered the principle that exercise must be vigorous enough to produce a sustained heart rate of 150 or more beats per minute. If it is not that vigorous, but is still demanding oxygen, it must be extended proportionately longer, depending on the oxygen consumed.

Before undertaking an aerobic exercise program you need some basic information. One good source is Dr. Cooper's book *The Aerobics Program for Total Well-Being.* A preliminary examination and clearance from your physician is important. You should begin gradually with a nontaxing level of activity. Monitoring your heartbeat by taking the pulse rate for 10-second intervals can assure you that you are not exceeding a safe level for your age and condition. If you feel excessively tired or develop pains in legs or chest, you should stop the program and see your doctor. These are common-sense precautions.

Exercise, then, is another area where we can make choices

that will improve our chances for a longer and better life. In this area of holistic health, perhaps as in no other, your choice is to be implemented, not contemplated. Someone else may be able to "feed you," but no one can "jog you" but you!

What Are You Living For?

What we are living for—our purpose in life—is a third vital area where our choices have an effect on wellness. Hope may be more essential to well-being than either nutrition or exercise. Whatever your age, if you are excited about your future, your body and mind respond positively.

Take the case of Sarah-Patton Boyle, who tells in her recent book, *The Desert Blooms,* how she lost her sense of purpose and how she recovered it. Her husband had left her, and her children were grown. She decided to move to Arlington, Virginia, and establish a new life for herself in the culturally rich environment of our nation's capital. Before long, however, she found that her dream of a totally free existence had become a nightmare of loneliness. Out of deep despair, with no hope of an answer, she prayed, "O God, help me!"

Nothing happened. She turned on the television set to break the silence and heard a man being interviewed on a talk show. He was describing the "serenity prayer" used by Alcoholics Anonymous. She clutched it, and her prayer for the courage to accept what she could not change was answered.

Looking herself in the eyes, she accepted that she was old, wrinkled, gray, defeated, tired, and lost. That radical act, as painful as it was, was the beginning of her healing. Her energy began to return.

She realized that her next step was to change the things

she could. She chose to start with herself. In the long list of her losses of the past five years, "the sense of progress" stood first. If she could recover that, she might regain a purpose for living.

Rejecting the notion that progress is not for old people, she resolved to acquire new attitudes, understandings, knowledge, and skills. She began by enrolling in a class in automobile mechanics. Then came study in philosophy, home economics, investments, psychology, and creative writing.

Slowly, painfully, but with peaks of joy and genuine satisfaction, she began to discover ways she could care for others and in that caring find fulfillment and purpose.

The theological word for what Patty Boyle lost and found is "hope." Hope is a gift of the God who calls us into a future that can be shaped by the choices we make. We are not prisoners of our past.

No matter what your present condition is—physically, mentally, morally, or spiritually—your future can be different. What you are living for exerts a powerful effect not only on your present attitude but ultimately upon your cells. Likewise, your choices today can play a powerful role in determining your wellness tomorrow. Why take chances when you can make choices?

How fearfully and wonderfully God has made us, mind and body! How caringly he has placed within us the powers that make for wellness. Wonder, awe, and reverence lead us to understand wellness as grounded in faith.

The wellness God promises is neither a prize for overachievers nor a reward for modern-day ascetics. In the final analysis, it is grace that makes us whole. We can do all the "right things" and not have perfect health, just as others can break all the rules and yet seem to remain well.

God's wholeness is more than physical and temporal. Even the most perfect bodies age and die. We can be permanently disabled, or even terminally ill, and still discover a wellness by opening ourselves to the love God pours into our hearts as his gift. How do we respond to the gift? The best response I know is the one Paul gave in Romans 12: "Present your bodies as a living sacrifice, holy and acceptable to God, which is your spiritual worship. Do not be conformed to this world but be transformed by the renewal of your mind, that you may prove what is the will of God, what is good and acceptable and perfect."

Appendix

The Social Readjustment Rating Scale

Life Event	Mean Value
1. Death of spouse	100
2. Divorce	73
3. Marital separation	65
4. Detention in jail or other institution	63
5. Death of a close family member	63
6. Major personal injury or illness	53
7. Marriage	50
8. Being fired at work	47
9. Marital reconciliation	45
10. Retirement from work	45
11. Major change in the health or behavior of a family member	44
12. Pregnancy	40
13. Sexual difficulties	39
14. Gaining a new family member (e.g., through birth, adoption, oldster moving in, etc.)	39
15. Major business readjustment (e.g., merger, reorganization, bankruptcy, etc.)	39
16. Major change in financial state (e.g., a lot worse off or a lot better off than usual)	38
17. Death of a close friend	37
18. Changing to a different line of work	36

Life Event	Mean Value
19. Major change in the number of arguments with spouse (e.g., either a lot more or a lot less than usual regarding childrearing, personal habits, etc.)	35
20. Taking out a mortgage or loan for a major purchase (e.g., for a home, business, etc.)	31
21. Foreclosure on a mortgage or loan	30
22. Major change in responsibilities at work (e.g., promotion, demotion, lateral transfer)	29
23. Son or daughter leaving home (e.g., marriage, attending college, etc.)	29
24. In-law troubles	29
25. Outstanding personal achievement	28
26. Wife beginning or ceasing work outside the home	26
27. Beginning or ceasing formal schooling	26
28. Major change in living conditions (e.g., building a new home, remodeling, deterioration of home or neighborhood)	25
29. Revision of personal habits (dress, manners, associations, etc.)	24
30. Troubles with the boss	23
31. Major change in working hours or conditions	20
32. Change in residence	20
33. Changing to a new school	20
34. Major change in usual type and/or amount of recreation	19
35. Major change in church activities (e.g., a lot more or a lot less than usual)	19
36. Major change in social activities (e.g., clubs, dancing, movies, visiting, etc.)	18
37. Taking out a mortgage or loan for a lesser purchase (e.g., for a car, TV, freezer, etc.)	17

Life Event	Mean Value
38. Major change in sleeping habits (a lot more or a lot less sleep, or change in part of day when asleep)	16
39. Major change in number of family get-togethers (e.g., a lot more or a lot less than usual)	15
40. Major change in eating habits (a lot more or a lot less food intake, or very different meal hours or surroundings)	15
41. Vacation	13
42. Christmas	12
43. Minor violations of the law (e.g., traffic tickets, jaywalking, disturbing the peace, etc.)	11

Questions for Thought and Discussion

1. What signs suggest an increased public interest in health?

2. Can health be adequately defined as freedom from disease?

3. Compare technological medicine with an ecological approach.

4. Name seven health practices that can increase average life expectancy seven to eleven years.

5. List the seven stages in the history of an illness.

6. Discuss the possible benefits and limitations of a health hazard appraisal.

7. What is implied by the Christian concept of the body as the temple of the Holy Spirit?

8. Suggest some ways in which our bodies "speak" to us.

9. Describe the process through which illness can lead to a redirection of one's life.

10. How can the destructive potential of "bad feelings" be averted?

11. What is your current score on the Holmes-Rahe Social Readjustment Rating Scale?

12. What new ways of managing and learning from stress have you considered?

13. List your personal goals for wellness.

14. List your major wellness resources: persons and groups.

15. What significant choices do you plan to make to support your personal wellness plan?

Suggestions for Further Reading

Ardell, Donald, and Tager, Mark J. *Planning for Wellness.* 2nd ed. Kendall/Hunt Publishing Co., 1982.

Ardrey, Robert. *The Social Contract.* Dell Publishing Co., 1970.

Boyle, Sarah-Patton. *The Desert Blooms: A Personal Adventure in Growing Old Creatively.* Abingdon Press, 1983.

Brand, Paul, and Yancey, Philip. *Fearfully and Wonderfully Made.* Zondervan Publishing House, 1980.

Chandler, Ted E. *How to Have Good Health.* Broadman Press, 1982.

Cooper, Kenneth H. *The Aerobics Program for Total Well-Being: Exercise, Diet, and Emotional Balance.* M. Evans, 1982.

Couey, Richard B. *Lifelong Fitness and Fulfillment.* Broadman Press, 1980.

Cousins, Norman. *Anatomy of an Illness As Perceived by the Patient.* W. W. Norton & Co., 1979.

———. *The Healing Heart: Antidotes to Panic and Helplessness.* W. W. Norton & Co., 1983.

Jaffe, Dennis T. *Healing from Within.* Bantam Books, 1982.

Larson, Bruce. *There's a Lot More to Health Than Not Being Sick.* Word Books, 1981.

Lynch, James J. *The Broken Heart: The Medical Consequences of Loneliness.* Harper & Row/Basic Books, 1979.

Pelletier, Kenneth R. *Holistic Medicine: From Stress to Optimum Health.* Delacorte Press/Seymour Lawrence, 1979.

Pilch, John J. *Wellness: Your Invitation to Full Life.* Winston Press, 1981.

Ratcliff, Lydia. *Health Hazard Appraisal.* Public Affairs Pamphlet No. 558.

Selye, Hans. *The Stress of Life.* McGraw-Hill Book Co., 1956.

Vaux, Kenneth L. *This Mortal Coil: The Meaning of Health and Disease.* Harper & Row, 1978.

Notes